The Every

excuse excuse excuse excuse excuse excuse excuse excuse
excuse excuse excuse excuse excuse excuse excuse excuse
excuse excuse excuse excuse excuse excuse excuse excuse
excuse excuse excuse excuse excuse excuse excuse excuse
excuse excuse excuse excuse excuse excuse excuse excuse
excuse excuse excuse excuse excuse excuse excuse excuse
excuse excuse excuse excuse excuse excuse excuse excuse
excuse excuse excuse excuse excuse excuse excuse excuse
excuse excuse excuse excuse excuse excuse excuse excuse
excuse excuse excuse excuse excuse excuse excuse excuse
excuse excuse excuse excuse excuse excuse excuse excuse
excuse excuse excuse excuse excuse excuse excuse excuse
excuse excuse excuse excuse excuse excuse excuse excuse
excuse excuse excuse excuse excuse excuse excuse excuse
excuse excuse excuse excuse excuse excuse excuse excuse

in the Book *Book*

A percentage of proceeds will go to the
Center for Celiac (Disease) Research.

The Every Excuse in the Book *Book*

How to Benefit from Exercising, by Overcoming Your Excuses

Jeanne "Bean" Murdock, owner
BEANFIT®

Illustrations by Bill Perry © 2005
Book design by Benjamin Lawless.
Set in Adobe Garamond Pro, Kenyan Coffee
and Adine Kirnburg Script.
Printed in the United States of America
by Ventura Printing
200 North Elevar Street
Oxnard, CA 93030

Library of Congress Control Number 2005905114
ISBN 0-9770678-0-7
EAN 9780977067800

ACKNOWLEDGEMENTS

A special thanks to Joe, not only for his encouragement and support, but also because he gave me quite a few of the excuses in this book. During his days of inconsistent workouts, he thought of so many creative alibis that I *had* to right them down. Then as I started paying attention to the reasons my clients gave me for not doing what I had asked of them, I realized I had a great idea for a book. I told Joe, "This is it! This is why many Americans are not exercising—they are making EXCUSES! I should write a book to illustrate why the excuses are invalid." He knew that I would do it, and assured me it would all work out. I thank him for always believing in me. I also thank my clients, even though I would rather that they'd exercised instead of made excuses.

Thank you to my friends and family, too, for their support and silence about what I was creating.

Thank you to Peter McWilliams for writing *Life 101: Everything We Wish We Had Learned About Life in School—but Didn't. Life 101* not only offered proverbs for my book, but also taught me a lot about life.

Thank you to the folks at K-Man Cyclery and Dale Pettit.

I dedicate this book to people who care about their health.

Table of Contents

Introduction 10

Excuses

Everything Else

Introduction

The clock ticks, approaching that magic hour—5:00! You're thinking, "Right after work, my **exercise** program commences. Goodbye, weight. Hello, waist line."

With fifteen seconds to go to freedom, the boss bellows, "By the way, there's a meeting after work today. I'll see you in 30 minutes."

"Damn! So much for the waist line. Who knows when I'll have time to exercise? Maybe it was a bad idea to think that I could proceed with a workout program at this stage of my life."

Does that sound familiar? Then this book is for you and every other person who permits other matters to supersede exercise.

How is this book different from any other exercise or motivational book? It lists 120 **excuses** not to exercise and explains why each one is invalid. This book also teaches you the importance of exercise, gets you motivated to start a program, and helps you be consistent and compliant for life. It should be read from cover to cover, so that you will have artillery to defend any excuse that attacks your conscience. Then you can use the book as reference: "I can't remember why Jeanne said that 'I hate exercising' is an invalid excuse."

* * *

We have heard time and time again the benefits of exercise, but nevertheless most Americans still don't do it. Why? You might think it's due to a lack of education about the benefits of exercise. I do not fall for that one. I am confident that it is due to EXCUSES. Most Americans seem to find other ways to use their time to avoid the dreaded task.

So why avoid exercise? Well, I know a lot of people who think that exercise is boring. So? What is the point? So is driving to work, but we do it. So is washing a car, but we make time for it to look good. Sitting under a salon hair dryer (I have done it once—I was in elementary school) is extremely boring, but people still choose to take care of their outsides more than their insides.

 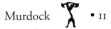

Just because something makes you uncomfortable, does not mean that you should automatically avoid it. For instance, remember getting a vaccination in your arm when you were young? Well, if you were like me, it made you uncomfortable, but you did not make an excuse to avoid it because the consequence could have been a crippling disease like **polio**. Maybe you would not be living now, if you had let your excuses overpower your knowledge to do what is right. The same thing can happen if you do not exercise. You could get a crippling disease like **osteoporosis** (brittle bones), or you could die at an early age from one of the top killers (listed from most to least prevalent)—**heart disease**, **stroke**, or **cancer**. Exercise can help prevent each of these maladies. If you think exercise makes you uncomfortable, think how much worse it would be to suffer from illness.

Refer to the glossary for definitions of terms in **this font**. Each vocabulary word will be in the special font just the first time that it appears in the book.

One more important note: Consult your physician, before starting an exercise conditioning program. The risks of exercising may include disorders of heartbeats, abnormal blood pressure response, and, very rarely, a heart attack.

* * *

Research overwhelmingly shows that regular exercise lowers the risk for many diseases, enhances the functioning of virtually every physiological system in the human body and improves psychological well-being. Unfortunately, fewer than 40 percent of Americans exercise enough to experience significant health benefits. As the following list indicates, 101 extraordinarily positive reasons* exist for you to exercise regularly. It is well-documented that exercise:

1. Helps you to more effectively manage **stress**.
2. Helps you to lose weight—especially fat weight.
3. Improves the functioning of your **immune system**.
4. Reduces medical and healthcare expenses.
5. Reduces your risk of getting heart disease.
6. Increases your level of muscle strength.
7. Improves athletic performance.
8. Can help relieve the pain of tension headaches—perhaps the most common type of headache.
9. Allows you to consume greater quantities of food and still maintain **caloric** balance.
10. Helps you sleep easier and better.
11. Enhances sexual desire, performance and satisfaction.
12. Reduces the risk of developing **hypertension** (high **blood pressure**).
13. Increases the density and breaking strength of bones.
14. Improves your physical appearance.
15. Increases circulating levels of **HDL** (good) **cholesterol**.
16. Assists in efforts to stop smoking.
17. Helps you to relax.

 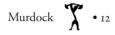

18. Can help improve short-term memory in older individuals.
19. Helps to maintain weight loss—unlike just **dieting**.
20. Helps relieve many of the common discomforts of pregnancy (backache, heartburn, constipation, etc.).
21. Reduces your anxiety level.
22. Helps control blood pressure in people with hypertension.
23. Protects against "creeping obesity" (the slow, but steady weight gain that occurs as you age).
24. Reduces your vulnerability to various cardiac dysrhythmias (abnormal heart rhythms).
25. Improves the likelihood of your survival from a **myocardial infarction**(heart attack).
26. Helps to overcome jet lag.
27. Slows the rate of joint degeneration in people with **osteoarthritis**.
28. Lowers your resting heart rate.
29. Helps to boost creativity.
30. Reduces your circulating levels of **triglycerides**.
31. Helps you resist upper **respiratory tract** infections.
32. Increases your **anaerobic threshold**, allowing you to work or exercise longer at a higher level, before a significant amount of **lactic acid** builds up.
33. Helps to preserve lean body tissue.
34. Improves your ability to recover from physical exertion.
35. Helps speed recovery from chemotherapy treatments.
36. Increases ability to supply blood to the skin for cooling.
37. Increases the thickness of the **cartilage** in your joints.
38. Gives you more energy to meet the demands of daily life, and provides you with a reserve to meet the demands of unexpected emergencies.
39. Increases your level of muscle endurance.
40. Helps prevent intestinal ulcers.
41. Increases the density and breaking strength of **ligaments** and **tendons**.
42. Improves posture.
43. Increases your **maximal oxygen uptake** ($\dot{V}O_2$ max—perhaps the best measure of your physical working capacity).
44. Helps you to maintain your **resting metabolic rate**.
45. Reduces the risk of developing **colon** cancer.
46. Increases your tissues' responsiveness to the actions of **insulin** (i.e., improves tissue sensitivity for insulin), which helps to better control blood sugar, particularly if you are a **type 2 diabetic**.
47. Helps to relieve constipation.
48. Expands **blood plasma** volume.
49. Reduces your risk of developing **prostate** cancer.
50. Helps to combat substance abuse.
51. Helps to alleviate depression.
52. Increases your ability to adapt to cold environments.
53. Helps you maintain proper muscle balance.
54. Reduces the rate and severity of medical complications associated with hypertension.
55. Helps to alleviate certain **menstrual** symptoms.
56. Lowers your heart rate response to submaximal physical exertion.

 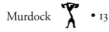

57. Helps to alleviate low-back pain.
58. Helps to reduce the amount of insulin required to control blood sugar levels in **type 1** (insulin-dependent) **diabetics.**
59. Improves mental alertness.
60. Improves respiratory muscle strength and muscle endurance—particularly important for **asthmatics.**
61. Reduces your risk of having a stroke.
62. Helps you to burn excess calories.
63. Increases your **cardiac reserve.**
64. Improves coronary (heart) circulation.
65. Offsets some of the negative side effects of certain antihypertensive drugs.
66. Increases your stroke volume (the amount of blood the heart pumps with each beat).
67. Improves your self-esteem.
68. Reduces your susceptibility of coronary thrombosis (a clot in an artery that supplies the heart with blood).
69. Reduces your risk of developing type 2 (non-insulin-dependent) diabetes.
70. Reduces the risk of developing breast cancer.
71. Improves mental cognition (a short-term effect only).
72. Maintains or improves joint flexibility.
73. Improves your **glucose tolerance.**
74. Reduces workdays missed due to illness.
75. Reduces the **viscosity** of your blood.
76. Enhances your muscles' ability to extract oxygen from your blood.
77. Increases your productivity at work.
78. Reduces your likelihood of developing low-back problems.
79. Improves your balance and coordination.
80. Improves your body's ability to use fat for energy during physical activity.
81. Provides protection against injury.
82. Decreases (by 20 to 30 percent) the need for antihypertensive medication, if you are a hypertensive.
83. Improves your decision-making abilities.
84. Helps reduce and prevent the immediate symptoms of menopause (hot flashes, sleep disturbances, irritability) and decrease the long-term risks of cardiovascular disease, osteoporosis and obesity.
85. Helps to relieve and prevent "migraine headache attacks."
86. Reduces the risk of **endometriosis** (a common cause of infertility).
87. Helps to retard bone loss as you age, thereby reducing your risk of developing osteoporosis.
88. Helps decrease your appetite (a short-term effect only).
89. Improves your pain tolerance and mood if you suffer from osteoarthritis.
90. Helps prevent and relieve the stresses that cause **carpal tunnel syndrome.**
91. Makes your heart a more efficient pump.
92. Helps to decrease left ventricular hypertrophy (a thickening of the walls of the left ventricle) in people with hypertension.
93. May be protective against the development of Alzheimer's disease.
94. Improves your mood.
95. Helps to increase your overall health awareness.

 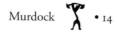

96. Reduces the risk of gastrointestinal bleeding.
97. Helps you to maintain an independent lifestyle.
98. Reduces the level of abdominal obesity—a significant health-risk factor.
99. Increases the diffusion capacity of the lungs, enhancing the exchange of oxygen from your lungs to your blood.
100. Improves heat tolerance.
101. Improves your overall quality of life.

*101 Reasons to Exercise in 2001

Copyright 2001, Fitness Management magazine, Leisure Publications Inc., Los Angeles, Calif., www.fitnessmanagement.com.

Additionally, you all have seen and heard about the hundreds of books and videotapes that show us the perfect workout, but even if there were such a thing, can the perfect workout encourage you to exercise? In most cases, no, because excuses are formed and exercise descends on the list of priorities. Certain illnesses are the only valid excuses for not exercising.

Unless you are ill frequently, here is what you can do to get around your excuses.

1. Understand why you make the excuses. One reason why you might make excuses is exercise makes you uncomfortable. You may be uncomfortable being seen in a gym or outside exercising. Whatever your excuses are, put them down on paper to learn more about yourself. When you have planned to exercise, but instead make an excuse, write down that reason. Think very carefully about it. The next time you plan to exercise and make an alibi instead, write down that excuse, too. Keep all of your excuses together on a piece of paper and compare them to each other. Is it always the same rationalization or are there a lot of different ones? Is there some sort of task that you have to take care of instead of exercising? Is it about how you feel that day? How important are these excuses? Asking yourself these questions and writing down the answers leads you to this lesson's second step.

2. Weigh the positive aspects of exercise to the positive aspects of your excuses. Verbalize your excuses and other thoughts, then read the benefits of exercise out loud (see the list on page 12). Which list truly speaks louder to you? The benefits of course.

3. Find ways to discard your excuses. This book contains a list of 120 excuses, which I heard while being a **personal fitness trainer**. The text below each excuse will assist you around an apparent problem, so that you can reap the benefits of exercise.

In some instances, it is simply not possible to do your planned regular workout, but that does not mean you should not exercise at all. It is a fact that losing weight is hard work, but it does not have to be grueling. It can be enjoyable. Imagine permanently discarding your excuses and exercising consistently and safely. You will never need to start a weight loss program again, and you will be so much healthier than you are now! When you have achieved your ideal weight, you will only need a maintenance program. Not only will the physiological effects of exercise make you feel better, but also the fact that you are doing it can elevate your self esteem (37).

 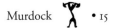

1

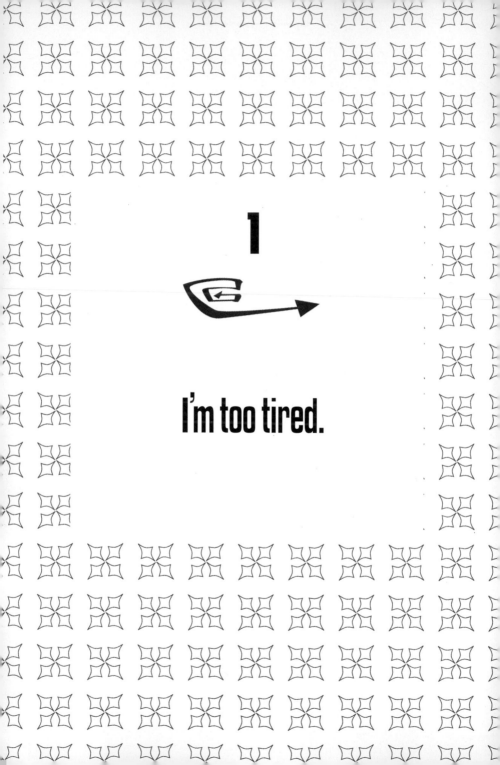

I'm too tired.

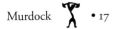

Exercise anyway. You probably will feel less tired afterwards. If you have been a sedentary person, exercise will probably make you more tired at first, but this will pass after a couple of months of consistently exercising. Your metabolic rate (speed of Calories burned) will increase, then the more you exercise, the less tired you will feel (unless you are overtraining), and the less you will be able to use this excuse.

Remember, the less you exercise the more tired you become, and the more tired you are the less apt you are to exercise. Break the vicious cycle by getting out today, even for a few minutes.

2

I'm too sore.

What part of you is sore? Is it your butt from doing squats? I have felt that soreness many times. It is smart not to work muscles that are sore, because they need more time to rest and repair. But you can still work parts of your body that are not sore. If your butt is sore, work on your upper body, or work your legs in ways that do not incorporate your gluteal (butt) muscles.

If your whole body feels sore, try walking slowly for a few minutes and then **stretching** well. Light exercise and stretching can make your muscles feel better by enhancing circulation.

 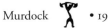

3

I don't have enough time.

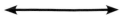

A German proverb states:

"Who begins too much accomplishes little."

You probably have time, but do not want to set some aside for exercise.

You need to take a serious look at your life and see what you find more important than your health. Maybe you need a time management course, too.

You don't have enough time, but you wait in long lines, wait "on hold" when making a phone call, wait for an elevator to arrive when you could be taking the stairs. You watch TV. You sit in traffic. You wait at the laundromat for your clothes to finish. You wait for your car to be finished at the local garage or car wash. You sit in a doctor's office. Maybe you hang out at the local bar and sit and visit with a friend? Why not exercise and talk with a friend?

Would you wait until your car conks out before doing a tune-up? Hopefully not. You would take care of it now, so that it could last you a long time.

Do not wait for your doctor to tell you—after he sees you for chest pains—to exercise. Exercise and eat properly now. Do not wait until you end up on high cholesterol and high blood pressure pills.

Be smart. MAKE time to exercise. Take care of yourself now, so that your body can last you a long time.

 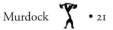

4

It's too hot out.

Go out and exercise anyway, but instead of going by yourself, bring a fan along.* It has been medically proven that pulling a fan burns more Calories than walking alone.

Seriously, try going for a walk in an air-conditioned mall.

Exercise early in the morning or late in the day. Remember ladies, go out with a buddy if it is dark outside. Wear light-colored clothes, so that other exercisers and cars can easily see you. In the daytime, wearing light-colored clothing can keep you cooler because they reflect the sun's rays. **Polypropylene**, or similar lightweight polyester, is a good choice of material for your clothes unlike silk and cotton, which retain moisture (17). To keep the sun off of your face, a visor is a better idea than a hat, because the hat can make your body retain heat.

To avoid **dehydration, heat exhaustion**, or **heatstroke** during exercise, drink cold fluids that are low in sugar concentration (less than 2.5 grams/100 ml of water). "Drink 13.5 to 20 ounces (two to three glasses) of the above drink thirty minutes before (exercising)," and about four to six ounces every 15 minutes during exercising, depending on the intensity of the workout (12). These amounts are in addition to the minimum eight 8-ounce glasses of water everyone should drink every day.

If you do choose to exercise outdoors instead of indoors, exercise at a lower intensity or less time than usual. Remember that something is better than nothing.

You can leave your air-conditioned house, drive in your air-conditioned car to an air-conditioned gym to exercise. If you do not have a gym membership, a lot of places will sell you a day pass. Most gyms will be more than happy to serve you, due to their normally decreased business in the summertime.

Or you can just stay home with that outdated aerobics videotape—led by an unqualified instructor—that you have always wanted to try. **JUST KIDDING**. Never follow exercise instruction from anyone who is an actress, model, bodybuilder, or professional athlete turned teacher. Make sure that the instructor is qualified, and has a degree in an exercise-related field. Rent or buy a video by Denise Austin or Kathy Smith.

*Do not try this. It is a joke.

5

It's too cold out.

Dress for it. "Start with long underwear made of polypropylene or a similar, lightweight polyester. Stay away from silk and cotton, which retain moisture. Next, layer with a synthetic fleece garment (Sanchilla and Polartec are two popular brands), followed by a breathable water and wind-resistant shell, such as rain pants and a windbreaker or rain jacket" (17). Wear mittens and polypropylene socks with a pair of wool socks over them (you may need slightly larger shoes to accommodate) (17). A warm hat is a must since at least 50% of body heat is lost through the head. A scarf around your neck would be good if your clothes do not go up that high, and a bandana around your mouth will help warm the air. Be careful not to over-layer. You will be warmer after you start exercising.

Start your workout slowly, since your joints will take a little longer to lubricate than if it were warm out.

Still be sure to drink fluid before and during the workout. Follow the guidelines expressed under excuse #4.

If you are determined not to go outside, exercise at home, in a gym, or in a heated mall.

 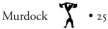

6

It's too wet out.

Remember that funny-looking yellow rain suit that you have seen city workers wearing in the winter; the same kind you said you'd never wear? Well, it is time to go out and invest in one. These days rubber rain suits come in more colors than yellow. Make sure that the jacket has a hood to keep your head warm and dry. Underneath the hood, you can wear a baseball hat to keep the rain off of your face, too. If you would rather take on the rain a little more stylishly, get an outfit made out of Gortex™.

Remember your feet. A pair of rubber boots or leather hiking boots treated with a waterproofing solution like Scotch Guard™ will keep your feet dry.

If it is not too wet out, just take along an umbrella and dress however you want.

If you are the type who does not like to be seen exercising outdoors, wet weather will be perfect for you. Few people are likely to be outside and you can disguise yourself in your rain gear.

Remember your other options — exercising in a mall, at home, or in a gym.

 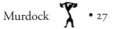

7

The gym was closed.

Oh, shoot. It is their fault that you can not exercise. Wrong! This is your chance to do something different. Go for a walk or hike in an area that you have always wanted to see. Rent roller skates (wear pads and a helmet) and use them where there are no cars. Pick up a new sport or re-play one that you have not tried in a while, but start slowly, because you may not be at the skill level that you expect.

Variety of exercise is just as important as doing it. Cross-training (doing different exercises or sports) stimulates and stresses the body positively. Cross-training works muscles you may not use in a single sport exercise program, and helps to prevent over-use injuries like **shin splints**, an idiopathic pain between the knee and the ankle. Regarding strength training, it is important to change your program every three months. This enables your muscles (and your mind) to stay stimulated and to avoid a plateau, where no physical or physiological changes occur.

If your gym is closed and you really want to get in some weight training, try to find one that is open. Otherwise, exercise at home.

 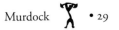

8

It's a holiday.

Even more reason to exercise. You have the day off, right? Great. Then, you will have more time. Maybe you can get in two workouts.

Oh, it is a religious holiday. I am sorry. I did not understand. Well, I know of no religion that says not to exercise on a particular day. If so, please prove me wrong. Besides, we choose to interpret religious teachings as we want and make some adjustments to suit our lifestyle.

Even God had to rest? Yes, but he had been exercising six days in a row. Have you? Furthermore, he only rested one day. Rest is a must. It is important to take off one day a week.

Often on holidays we tend to eat a little more than usual. Try exercising before your big meal. Since exercise increases your metabolism and keeps it elevated even hours afterwards (depending on length and intensity of session), it will be more likely that your food will be digested properly and used as energy rather than stored as fat. "Walking off" your meal is a bad idea. When you exercise, blood is **shunted** to the working muscles and away from the stomach, which can result in indigestion and even a **side stitch** (cramp in your side). The best thing to do after eating is to sit. Your food will digest better than if you lie down. If you are determined to lie down, lie on you left side to help prevent **reflux** (heartburn).

 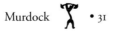

9

I'm on vacation.

Since you treated yourself to a vacation, treat yourself to exercise, too.

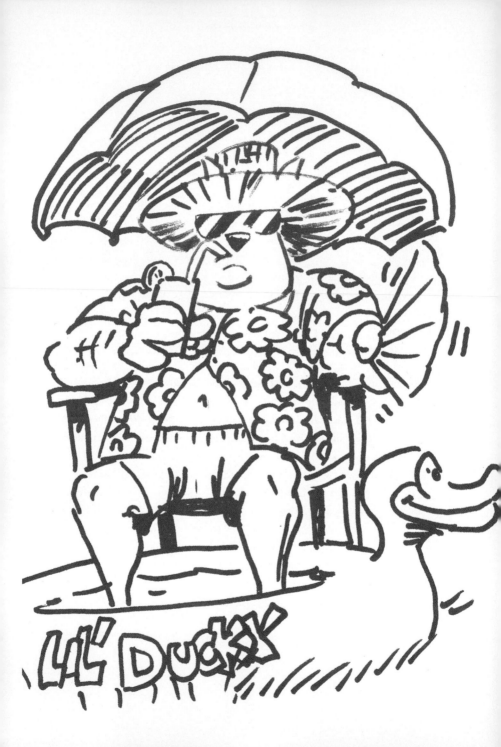

Since you treated yourself to a vacation, treat yourself to exercise, too. This is a great time to exercise. You have more time on your hands than usual and no work or prior commitments to which to attend.

If you go away from home for vacation and stay in a hotel, choose a place with a gym, pool, or tennis court or other exercise facilities. It does not take much of a break from exercise to lead you right back to where you started physically. It is a lot of hard work to achieve results, so maintain them. If there are no facilities where you are staying, just exercise in your room.

Nowadays it is not too hard to find a gym. Just tell the gym manager you are visiting the area and you would like to get a temporary pass. Also, find out if your gym membership at home can transfer to gyms in other areas.

Plan a vacation where you get to sightsee by bike or other exercise mode. Backpacking, horseback riding, and kayaking trips are available, too, by many outdoor companies—ask your travel agent. Plan to walk as much as possible, instead of taking cabs, trolleys, or rental cars in downtown areas.

Consider going on a cruise. Many cruise ships have exercise programs throughout each day. Read the company's brochure or call for a schedule of workouts, so that you will know what to pack.

If you had not been exercising before vacation, you might want to spend your days at a spa. This is a great way to start exercising for life! Be careful, though. Exercise at your own level, not so hard that after your trip you have to spend all your time resting. Spas are great places to learn how to live healthier lifestyles and even kick nasty habits like smoking. Beware of the Caloric intake that you are allowed each day. Some spas go dangerously low (below 1200 Calories per day). Find out before you make a reservation.

 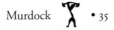

10

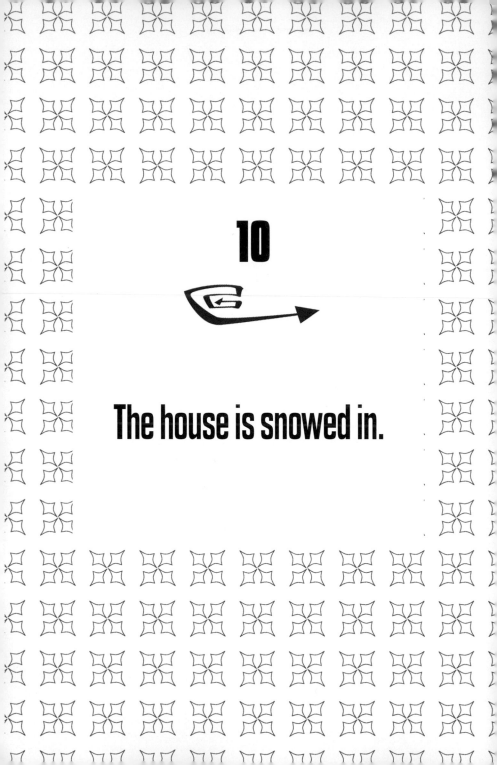

The house is snowed in.

Time to start shoveling! Not only is shoveling snow a great form of exercise, but also you will be able to clear the path from the door to go outside and exercise further. Keep in mind, though, that since shoveling is exercise, you should work with frequent breaks, if you are unfit.

You can also stay home and exercise. Find some chores to do around the house. Cleaning, repairing, and maintaining your house is a good way to stay active while stuck at home.

Put on some of your favorite music and start dancing. It does not matter which type of dancing you choose (although, the more rigorous types burn more Calories), just as long as you **MOVE**.

If you have a child, try doing everything that he does (like playing follow the leader), instead of just trying to contain him. That provides a great indoor workout.

Do you have stairs in your home? Start climbing. Walk or run up each step and slowly walk down each step. When you slowly walk down stairs (or a hill), your muscles have to work harder since they are fighting gravity. Also, it is easier on your joints.

 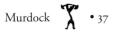

11

I'm on a business trip.

See if your associates will discuss business while walking. It is not so far fetched; exercise stimulates the thought process. I challenge you to ask. You can still bring a note pad and pen to take notes, if necessary. You do not have to exercise during your whole discussion.

Nowadays a lot of hotels have exercise rooms. Make a point to stay at such a place. If there is no fitness facility, walk up and down the building's stairs a few times.

Find a gym in the area and get a week or day pass.

It is important to continue exercising when you are away on business because it will help you manage stress, prevent jet lag, and maintain your fitness level. Take advantage of meeting breaks. Find some stairs to climb or just walk around the office.

 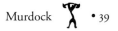

12

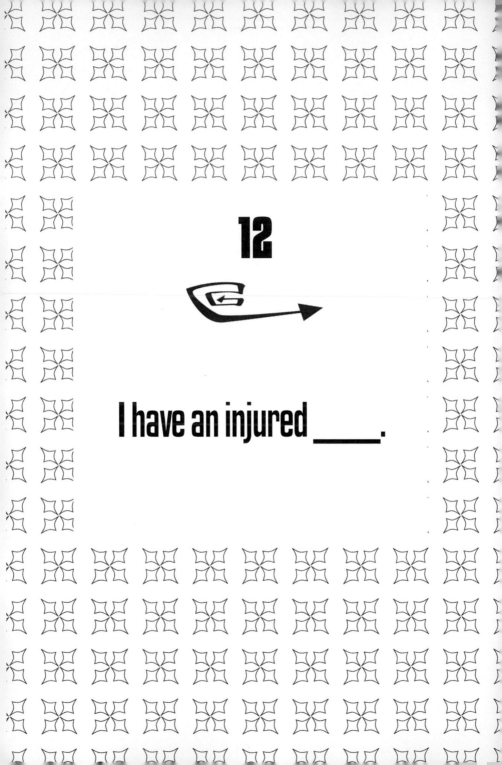

I have an injured ____.

Exercise whatever parts are still healthy. If you have an injured arm, you can still do **cardiovascular exercise** that involves just your legs. Using **dumbbells**, **strength train** the uninjured arm. Not only will you keep the healthy arm fit, but also you will help preserve the muscle in the injured arm. Research suggests that there is stimulation (bilateral transfer) in a sedentary limb, when the opposite (contralateral) limb is being exercised (6,14,16,23,28,31).

If you have an injured leg, strength train your upper body and the uninjured leg. Bilateral transfer applies to the legs, too.

If you are not wearing a cast and you can get your injured limb wet, consider water exercises, especially if you can not stand on a leg. Invest in an AquaJogger™ and a good aquatic exercise book (24).

If you have a broken bone, a strained muscle or tendon, or a sprained ligament, get physical therapy. Getting professional rehabilitation will help you heal properly and help prevent re-injury and osteoarthritis. It is very common to re-injure a ligament, muscle, or tendon. Sometimes they are left weak after the first trauma because they do not heal properly.

 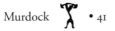

13

I can't afford to.

J. P. Donleavy said:

"When you don't have any money, the problem is food. When you have money it's sex. When you have both it's health. If everything is simply jake, then you're frightened of death."

Do you know how much it costs to have heart surgery? Thousands of dollars! Do you know how much it costs to buy a pair of walking shoes? Maybe $40, if you want them to last. Compare the figures. Would you rather spend all of your hard-earned money on surgery or athletic equipment? Walking and other aerobic exercise help prevent cardiovascular disease (3).

If you cannot afford a gym membership, a leotard, and Chanel No. 5™, it is OK. Work with what you have.

If you have a few extra dollars, invest in some equipment for your home. You do not have to get a $3000.00 machine, just start with some dumbbells or even a Dynaband™. See if a friend wants to help pay for or share some exercise equipment with you.

You might get a discount at a gym, if you bring a friend along with you.

Not only does your time need to be budgeted well to allow for exercise, but also your pocket book. All good budgets allow for some flexibility. Look at what you are buying and decide if it is really more important than your health. If you do not have a budget, now is a good time to start managing your money well.

Do not let money get in the way of exercising. If you do not exercise now, you will literally pay for it later. All of the bills will eventually pile up for illnesses that could have been prevented by exercising.

 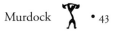

14

I'm too old.

Socrates said:

"The only good is knowledge and the only evil is ignorance."

Too old? Those of you who think that you are too old to start exercising probably think that you are too old to get a disease, too. Think again. Anyone who can move can do some sort of exercise. As for diseases, anyone can get one—especially those diseases often related to lifestyle: heart disease, cancer, stroke, diabetes, and osteoporosis, among others.

Exercise is not only for body builders and models, but also for those who want to maintain the capacity for independent living, reduce the risk of heart disease, slow the progression of chronic diseases, promote mental wellness, and socially interact. The proper exercise program can help you overcome the limitations that come with age, and yield a healthy lifestyle.

According to the American College of Sports Medicine (ACSM), precautions should be taken with certain individuals before starting an exercise program. A medical exam and diagnostic exercise test is recommended for:

- apparently healthy men over 40 and women over 50 years old who want to start a vigorous (intense enough to cause fatigue in 20 minutes) exercise program;
- **asymptomatic**, higher risk (e.g., a smoker) people who want to start a vigorous exercise program; and
- any higher risk, symptomatic (e.g., chest pains) person or one with disease (cardiac, **pulmonary**, or metabolic) who wants to start any type of exercise program.

Physician supervision is recommended during exercise testing for:

- men over 40 and women over 50 years old who will have maximal (exercising until exhaustion) testing;
- asymptomatic, higher risk individuals who will have maximal testing; and
- a higher risk, symptomatic person or one with disease who will have submaximal or maximal testing (3).

Regarding the exercise program itself, it should be individualized according to the results of exercise testing (if done) and specific needs of the participant. "Walking, chair and floor exercises, and modified strength/flexibility calisthenics are well-tolerated by most elderly individuals. Water exercise (24), swimming or cycling may be more appropriate for those with bone/joint problems" (3).

 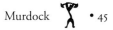

15

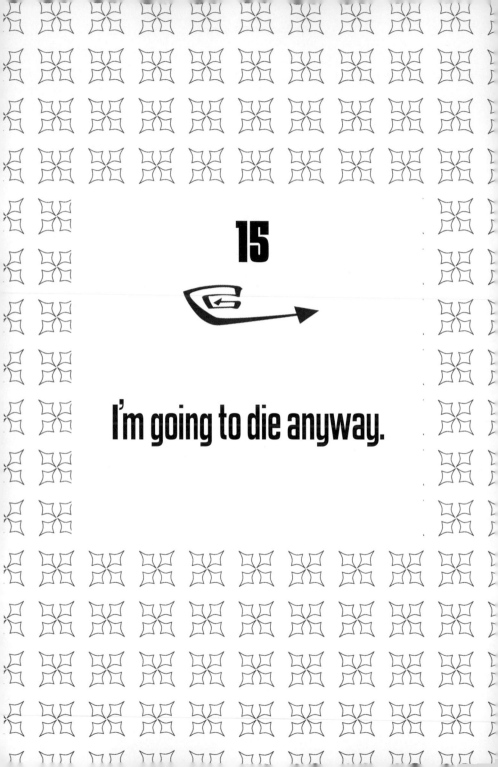

I'm going to die anyway.

Lily Tomlin said:

"No matter how cynical you get, it is impossible to keep up."

Would you rather die in your sleep at age 90 after living a healthy, disease-free life, or age 49 after battling cancer for five years? Suffering is no fun. I speak from experience in that I have seen people suffer from preventable diseases. Take my dad, for example. He ate poorly, never exercised, smoked three packs of cigarettes a day, was always stressed, and drank a six-pack of beer a night. Somehow, he had very low blood pressure and cholesterol, but nevertheless died at age 59 from prostate cancer. He suffered for three years, spending all of his time either at the hospital for treatments or at home—too weak to go out. Although prostate cancer is often inherited and is highly treatable, his lifestyle not only led him toward destruction, but also accelerated the disease's progression.

People tend to forget that in addition to mortality, they should consider morbidity—the length of time one will suffer before dying. Only some "lucky" ones die suddenly. Would you really want to die suddenly without the chance of saying, "Goodbye," or without accomplishing one more goal?

Also, people argue that if they are extremely sick, "Just pull the plug." Do you know how difficult it is to "pull the plug" in the United States? It can take years of legal processes for a family member to accomplish such a wish.

Do not be a victim of your unhealthy lifestyle. If you have a lot of bad habits, make a point to change them. Not all need to change at once. Set realistic goals. Have exercise be the first habit you establish. It is very likely that once you start an exercise program you will feel so good that any other bad habits will eventually fade away. It is amazing how the natural high can sway you to make healthier choices.

 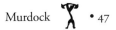

16

It's too much trouble.

Carl Jung said:

"Nobody, as long as he moves about among the chaotic currents of life, is without trouble."

How hard is it to walk out the door and around the block a few times? Exercise does not have to be an arduous task. You do not have to do your hair nicely or wear a fancy outfit. Even if you choose to make it an arduous task, it doesn't matter. At least you are doing it. But, be realistic. If you are making exercise a chore, you probably will not stick with the program.

If you are using this excuse, you probably will not choose swimming for your exercise or working out during a lunch break where you would have to change your clothes twice. Try a walking program so you will only need special shoes. Walking can be done anywhere at anytime and it is free!

Do not make exercise more difficult than it is. Set realistic goals and plan well so that exercise doesn't seem like a lot of trouble. After being on a program for a few months, you will start noticing results and be proud of yourself for making the time to exercise. Feeling healthy is not too much trouble, is it?

17

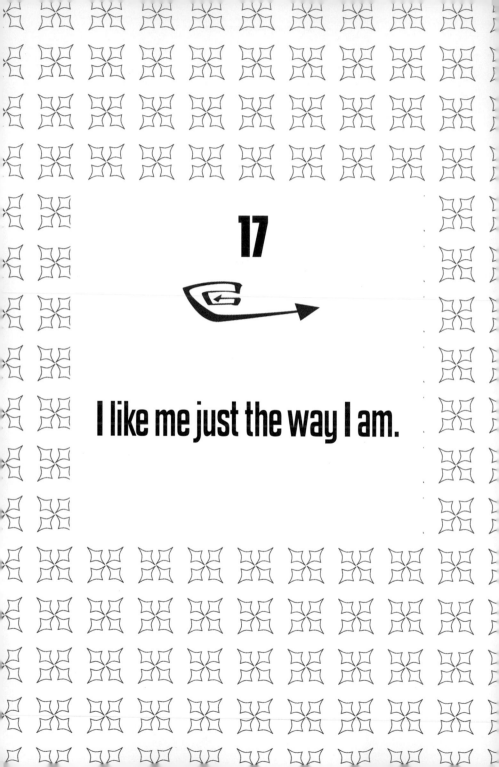

I like me just the way I am.

Keep fooling yourself. It is important to love yourself no matter what, but you do not have to like how you look or feel. Do you like feeling sluggish, growing out of clothes, being exhausted after walking a flight of stairs, and being at risk for several **obesity**-related diseases like diabetes? Even if you feel fine, you do not know how much better you can feel until you start exercising. You might realize that you lacked energy and really were not happy with how you looked. You may feel fine now, but if you are obese and you do not exercise consistently, you may as well plan for having a lifestyle-related problem like heart disease. The odds are against you.

You may be thin, eat anything you want and not gain weight, and like yourself just the way you are, but you have to exercise, too. A thin person may look fine on the outside, but not be healthy on the inside. Exercise can increase HDL (good) cholesterol, which can help prevent atherosclerosis (clogging of the arteries). Yes, even thin people may have atherosclerosis, hypertension (high blood pressure), and hypercholesterolemia (high cholesterol), all of which can be improved with exercise.

If you are afraid changing the way you are will lead to needing a whole new wardrobe, do not worry. If you are thin, the right exercise can not only bring little change in your size, but also make you healthier. If you are obese, so what if you lose weight and have to get new clothes? You will get to add quality to your closet and your life!

I remember Oprah Winfrey using this excuse when she gained all of her weight back, plus some, after her second to last effort to lose weight. I just about fainted when I heard it, because I knew that she had a lot of followers watching her every move. I imagined all of the obese people hearing her and starting to think the same thing. Then they too would give up on their health just like she had done. Fortunately it was temporary and she was motivated to give it another try—successfully! She was successful, because she did it safely and effectively by eating properly and exercising instead of dieting. Yeah for Oprah! I applaud her for trying hard and being a good role model.

 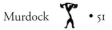

18

It's too hard.

Make it easier, then. Exercise does not have to be intense when you first get started. As a matter of fact, making your workout more intense than it needs to be will make you not want to exercise, or make you very sore or create injury.

ACSM publishes a book (3) of exercise testing and prescription guidelines. This book is the "bible" for us fitness professionals (unfortunately, not enough use it). ACSM recommends exercising five times a week, 30 minutes, which can be divided into two 15-minute intervals, each day. Even at a moderate intensity, exercise helps prevent heart disease and decreases body fat. More intense workouts enhance the benefits of exercising, but you should progress slowly, especially if you are obese (women—more than 30% body fat; men—more than 25%). In addition to walking, swimming, and weight training, activities that count as exercise include house cleaning, gardening, and stair climbing.

 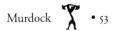

19

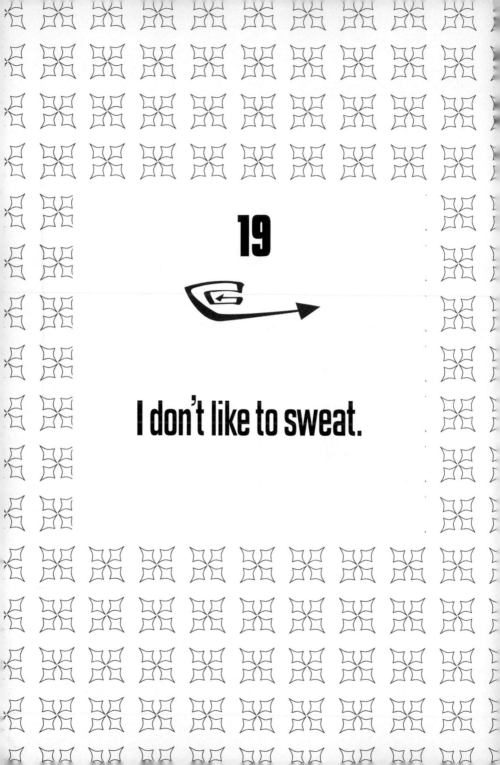

I don't like to sweat.

The more trained you are the more likely you are to sweat, because your cooling system becomes more efficient.

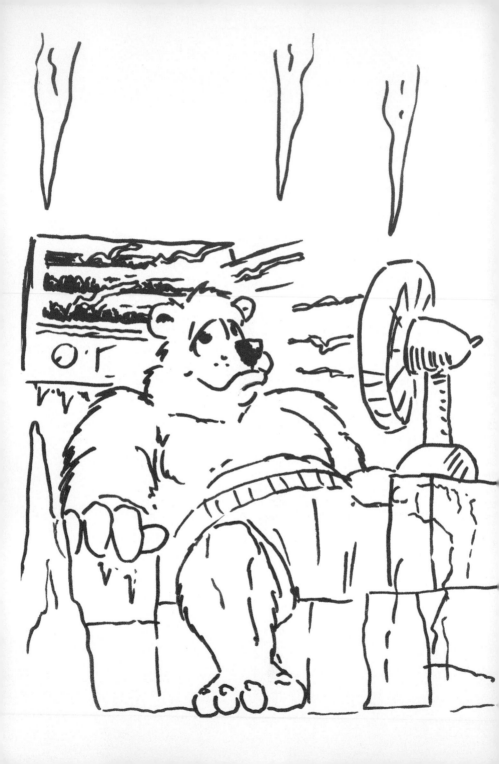

Well like it or not everyone sweats—everyday—with or without exercising. It is one of the body's ways of regulating its core temperature. Sweating is especially essential during exercise. As the duration of exercise lengthens, more heat is produced from the Calories burned.

To help your body stay cool, wear special clothing. If you are indoors, do not wear a hat, since approximately 50% of lost body heat goes through the head. Wear shorts and a lightweight shirt. Wear a visor and lightweight, light-colored clothes, if you are outdoors in the sun exercising (see #4).

Get used to sweating. The more trained you are the more likely you are to sweat, because your cooling system becomes more efficient. Women and men sweat at about the same rate, but a woman's body will reach one degree higher than a man's before starting to sweat (42). In mild hyperthermia (body temperature rises one to two degrees), exercise performance can be affected by a hyper-increased heart rate and decreased muscular function. If the body temperature rises to 105° or 106° F, neurological damage and death can occur.

 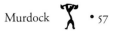

20

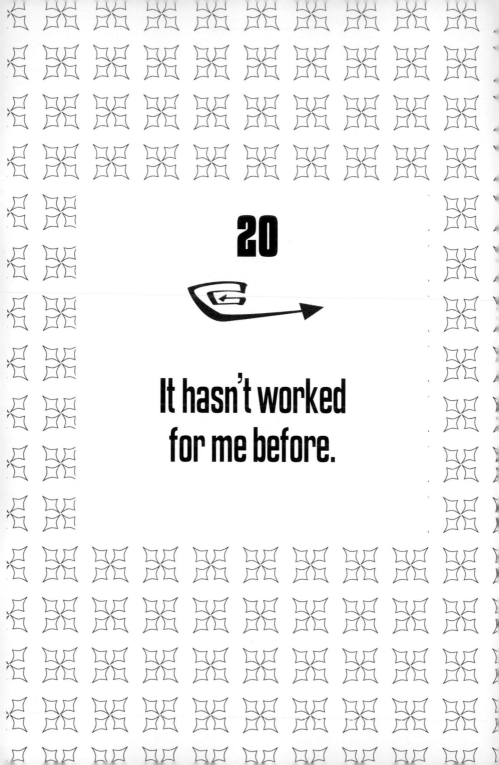

It hasn't worked
for me before.

Are you still exercising? That is why it has not worked for you. Exercise needs to be performed consistently to lose weight and to keep the weight off. If you are exercising properly, you should start noticing changes after about three months. It takes about eight to twelve weeks for changes at the cellular level, before fat is oxidized (burned) more efficiently and muscle is built.

At the beginning of your program, you will burn some fat during exercise, but it can take up to three months before a significant amount is withdrawn from your fat cells and used for energy. Then, you will notice more fat loss. Eventually, the rate at which you lose fat decreases. Do not be alarmed. If you are exercising properly you will continue to lose fat. However, you may need to change your program every three months or so to make sure that you keep your body stimulated enough not to hit a plateau.

It is common to hit a weight plateau. This happens when the body reaches its set point, which is theorized to be the body's desired weight. You can get off of the plateau or prevent it, by changing the program or increasing the exercise volume. Eventually there will be a final plateau, but continue until that weight or body composition is a healthy one. Continue exercising to maintain it.

 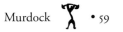

21

I'm just going to diet.

Diets don't work.

Diets cause the body to go into a starvation mode. This means that your metabolism decreases, because your body knows it is not getting enough food and it wants to conserve energy. Your body then uses some of its stored energy to stay alive. This may not only result in a loss of fat, but also muscle (including the heart muscle), which yields protein for energy.

When muscle mass is lost, the metabolism slows further due to the fact that there is less muscle to burn Calories. Keep in mind that to sustain itself, muscle burns more Calories than fat tissue.

If a decrease in weight is noticed at the beginning of a diet, it is most likely due to water loss. This excess water excretion is from the breakdown of glycogen (stored carbohydrate) to glucose (blood sugar—readily available energy). Later, weight loss is probably due to loss of muscle mass and should not be applauded. "With prolonged Caloric restriction, however, water can be retained on occasion to the point that it may cause weight gain even though fat and protein losses continue" (7).

When normal Caloric intake is resumed (after dieting), the body is quick to store (especially as fat) the extra Calories it obtains. One reason is that it wants to be prepared for the next fast, and the other reason is that it does not need as many Calories as it did before the diet because the metabolism is slower. The final result is less muscle, more fat, and more weight than before the diet.

Healthy eating habits are important, but visiting diet centers, taking pills and powders, and drinking liquid meals are not the solution. They are unhealthy choices and cause more damage than good. Even Nutri System® had 18 people from Florida file a lawsuit against them, claiming the program caused gallstones (32).

 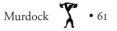

22

It didn't help my friend.

Exercise affects everybody differently. If you are obese and have a history of **yo-yo dieting** you will have a more difficult time losing weight than people who never diet. The dieter's body is more resistant to change, assuming that it might experience another famine. An obese person also has a lot more weight to lose than a thinner person, and probably has a slower metabolism at the start of an exercise program. These two disadvantages mean that it will take a while for an obese person to reach her goal, which requires a lot of patience. The wait is worthwhile, though!

There may be other reasons why exercise did not help your friend. Is your friend still exercising? No? Exercise can't help one to lose weight if it is not done. Yes, your friend is still exercising? It can take eight to twelve weeks from the start of a program, before fat starts to oxidize (burn) at a greater rate than normal. During the following few months fat loss will be more apparent. Later the rate of fat loss slows considerably, and may even stop if the exercise program is not changed and the volume is not increased. Variety is important, because the muscles, as well as the mind, get bored with the same workout. Without periodic adjustments to your routine you will hit a plateau, which means that your body will stop improving.

An exercise program becomes ineffective, when performed improperly or designed incorrectly. Consult a personal fitness trainer to ensure that you are using proper form and doing the correct intensity, duration, mode, and frequency—level of work, length of time, type, and occasions per week, respectively.

In one week you must burn 3500 Calories more than you consume to lose a pound of fat that week. If you have an appropriate workout, but still eat too much, you will not lose weight. Eating properly complements an exercise program.

It is possible that your friend was not losing weight per se, but was favorably changing his body composition. He could have gained muscle mass and lost fat, thereby lowering his percentage of body fat, without changing his weight. Even if more pounds of fat are lost than muscle gained, total body weight may stay the same, because muscle weighs more than fat, and takes up 1/3 the space (pound for pound) of fat.

 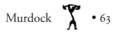

23

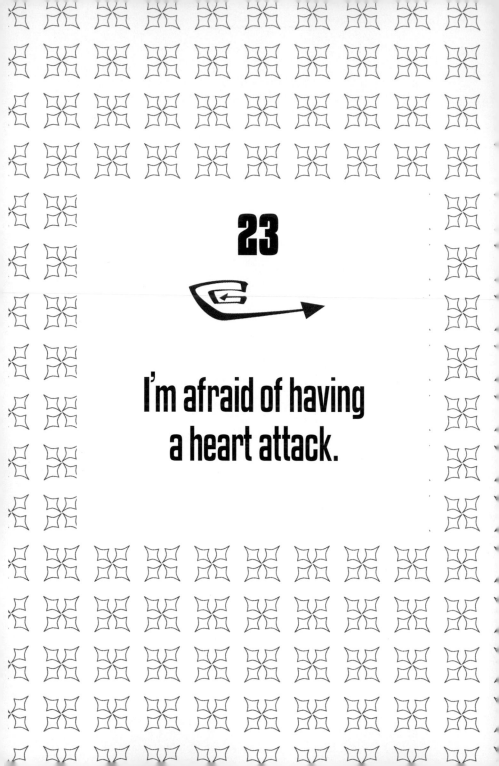

I'm afraid of having a heart attack.

Mel Brooks stated:

Look, I really don't want to wax philosophic; but I will say that if you're alive, you got to flap your arms and legs, you got to jump around a lot, you got to make a lot of noise, because life is the very opposite of death. And therefore, as I see it, if you're quiet, you're not living. You've got to be noisy, or at least your thoughts should be noisy and colorful and lively.

Yes, it is possible that exercise will induce a heart attack. If your heart is that sick, any stress (positive or negative) can spark a heart attack.

Before starting an exercise program, get a physical examination from your physician. If you are especially concerned, you can have a stress test to see if there is any unusual heart activity while you are exercising. A stress test usually involves being hooked up to an EKG (electrocardiogram) monitor while on a treadmill. It is not predetermined exactly how long you will be on the treadmill. It depends what your heart rate, blood pressure, and heart responses are during the test. Stress tests are nothing to be afraid of, and are designed especially to your fitness level. After the session, your doctor will tell you whether the test was negative (no unusual heart activity) or positive (unusual heart activity), and then may give you approval to start an exercise program.

Even if you get approval, start slowly. Give your body time to adapt to the exercise you choose. Later, you can increase the volume. Also, remember a heart attack is most likely to occur in the weekend warriors than in those who exercise consistently.

Furthermore, to reduce your risk for heart disease, avoid smoking, eat properly, and keep your cholesterol and blood pressure levels low. If you do not know the latter two levels, find out. Normal cholesterol level is below 200 mg/dl (milligrams/deciliter) of blood and normal blood pressure is below 140/90 mm/Hg (millimeters of mercury).

One last word on this topic. The name Jim Fixx (a former exercise guru and runner) often comes to mind when talking about exercise and heart attack. Jim Fixx had a rare heart defect and probably would have died young no matter how much he exercised. Running did not cause his early demise.

 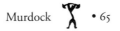

24

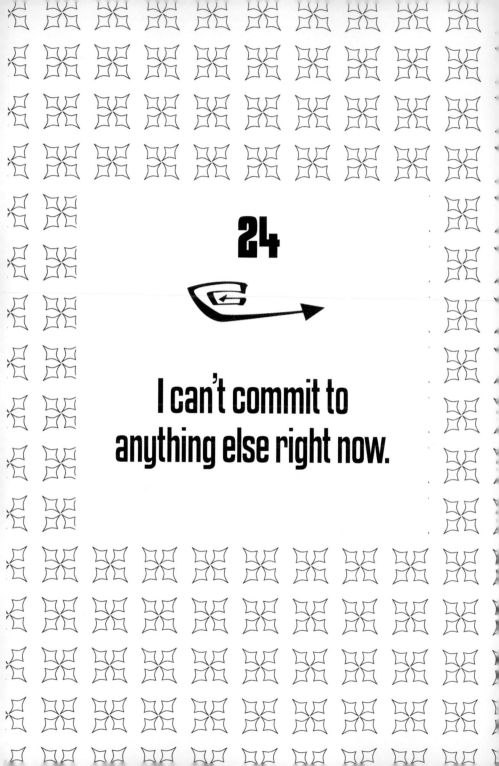

I can't commit to anything else right now.

H. L. Hunt stated:

"Decide what you want, decide what you are willing to exchange for it. Establish your priorities and go to work."

It is time to review your priorities, then. Also, you need a time management class. What do you think is more important than exercise?

At some point we do need to say no to excessive commitments, but don't say no to exercise. It does not need to take up all of your time—only 30 minutes five times a week. The 30 minutes can be divided into two 15-minute sessions.

You do not even have 15 minutes to set aside? You probably are the type of person, then, who does not do anything for himself and will die at an early age. If you want to live a long, healthy life, start taking time away from your responsibilities to care for yourself. You are one of your responsibilities.

Start by making a list of all of the things you need to do, including work if employed. Then, number them according to their importance—exercise should be number one! When enumerating, consider that some things can be delegated to others, such as cleaning, yardwork, laundry, and errands. It is amazing how many businesses will come to your home, nowadays, to serve you. Think about hiring a maid, gardener, or neighbor kid to do things that *you* do not have to do. If you have a family, be sure to delegate chores to everyone.

Do not try to be superman or superwoman. It is OK if you do not do everything yourself. Then while you are taking time out for yourself, you will be grateful that you delegated. You will have time to exercise, and will be healthier, and less stressed.

25

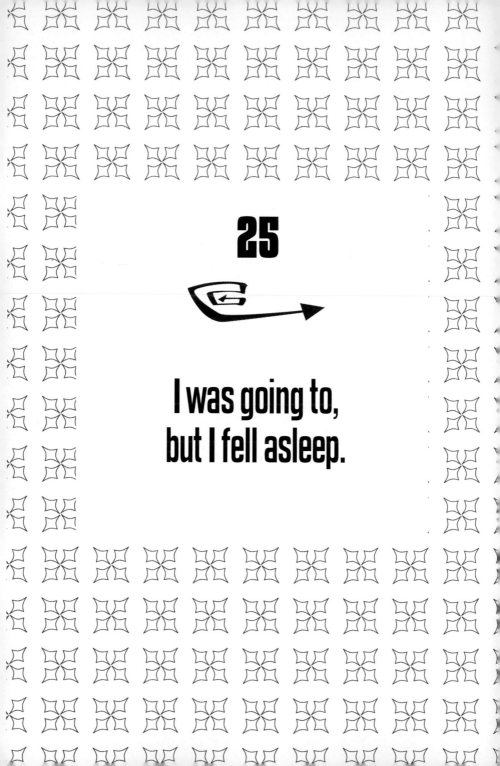

I was going to,
but I fell asleep.

Exercise gives you energy. How many times have you heard that? It is true. If you exercise regularly, you will have more energy and will not have as much trouble staying awake.

If you have this problem at night, plan to exercise in the morning. You probably will have more energy during the day.

If you fall asleep in the middle of the day, then exercise when you awaken. Do whatever you have to in order to exercise.

If you slept while you were supposed to be at an exercise class, then just do something on your own now.

 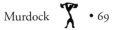

26

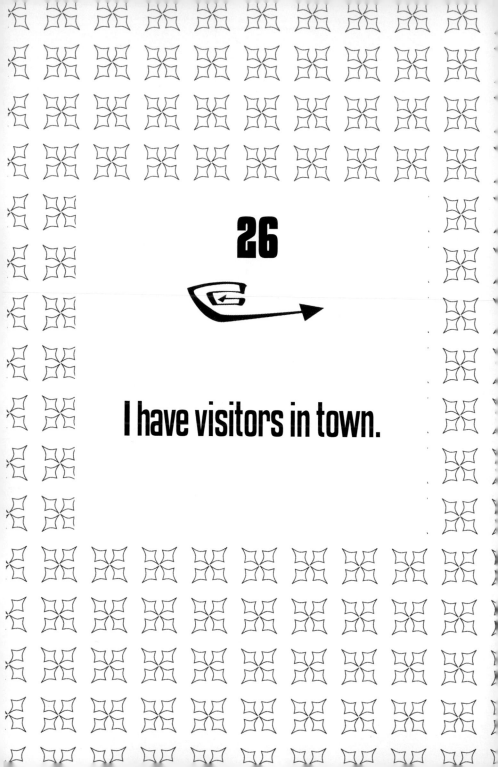

I have visitors in town.

Perfect. Take them with you to workout. A lot of gyms offer members free guest passes and on-site personal fitness trainers to teach new people how to use the equipment.

Walking provides a great time for catching up with visitors and allows quality time without distractions like phone calls, door-to-door salesmen, and the television.

Plan a walking tour of the town or downtown area for newcomers. Look into available walking, hiking, or biking tours in the vicinity.

If the visitors had not been exercising consistently, it will be a great chance for them to start! If they had been exercising they will appreciate staying active while they are away from home. Plus, they won't be able to use excuse #9!

Plan other exercise-related activities to keep the guests entertained, such as water sports, ice skating, roller skating, horseback riding, golfing (walking the course), and tennis.

 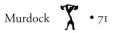

27

I just got home from work
and can't get myself
out, again.

Try using a forklift.* Come on. You can get yourself out, again. You just don't want to. Think about how much better you will feel, emotionally and physically, if you exercise. If you do not exercise when you had planned to, this excuse will become more of a habit than exercise. The next thing you know, you will be right back where you had started. "For every 72 hours you're idle, you lose 5% of your acquired strength" (36).

Try going straight from work to the gym, park, or wherever you exercise, instead of going home first. Leave your house in the morning with a change of clothes and a healthy snack to have after work (before you exercise). If you have to go home first, do not sit down; it is too hard to get back up, again.

If you were planning on exercising outdoors, just do it where you work. Bring your bike, walking shoes, or skates. Work, then do your workout, then you can go home.

*Do not try this. It is a joke.

 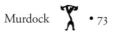

28

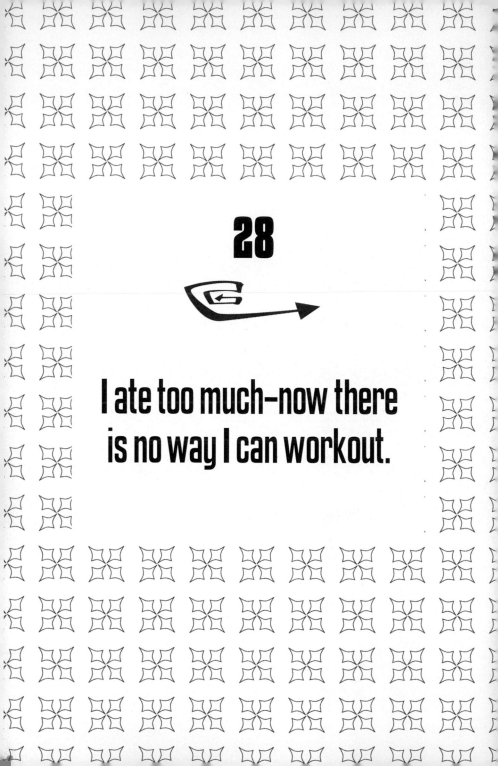

I ate too much—now there is no way I can workout.

Allow your body two or three hours to digest some of the food, and then workout at a comfortable intensity.

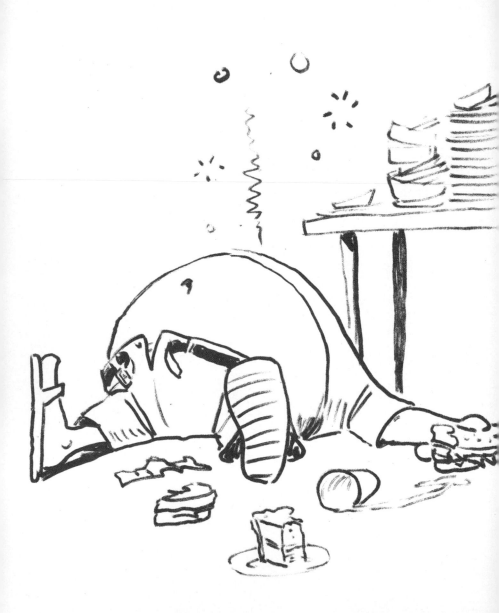

Plan to exercise **before** you eat. Your metabolism will be higher and there will be less chance that what you eat will be stored as fat than if you had not exercised at all.

The so-called walking-off-a-meal program is not a good one. The best thing to do after eating a meal is to sit. Sitting is better than lying down, because it helps prevent reflux. Because of how your stomach is shaped, lying on your left side rather than right will decrease the chance of reflux, if you must lie down. When you exercise after eating a meal, the working muscles compete with the digestive system for blood. As a result, you might incur indigestion, a side stitch, or early muscle fatigue.

It is OK to eat before exercising, if you consume a snack or small meal.

If you eat too much, allow your body two or three hours to digest some of the food, and then workout at a comfortable intensity. Otherwise, make up for lost exercise time tomorrow.

 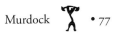

29

I can't get psyched up for it.

Will the words obesity, cardiovascular disease, cancer, diabetes, muscle atrophy (loss), and osteoporosis help? You do not have to get psyched up for those to occur. In fact they occur without much effort at all.

Put in the effort. The longer you try to get psyched up for it, the more time you will have to find other excuses. Then the next thing you know, you are spending all of your time re-reading this book (not to undermine its importance), when you could be performing your workout.

You know that you will feel a lot better when you are done exercising. Just go.

 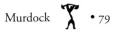

30

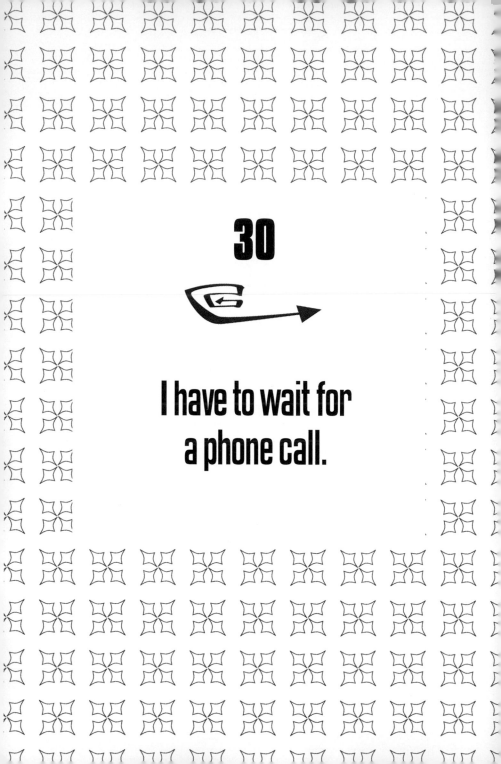

I have to wait for a phone call.

Take your phone with you. If you use this excuse a lot, it is time to buy a mobile phone. Add up all of the time that you spend just sitting around waiting for a phone call then multiply it by the value of your time. I bet that you will find it is less than the value of a mobile phone.* That time can not only be spent exercising, but also earning money.

If I ever have to leave the house when someone is supposed to call me, I just call him and say: "I would have waited for you to call, but I need to get going. Can we talk now or should I call you back later?"

When people call you back later than they say they will, tell them that you were disappointed that they did not call on time. Do not be afraid to tell them, otherwise it will happen again.

Alternatively, you can exercise at home while you are waiting for the phone to ring. Put on some music and dance, climb up and down your stairs if you have them, clean, or get warmed up for your workout by jogging or walking in place for five minutes, then stretching.

*Some studies suggest that mobile phone radiation is harmful.

 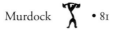

31

I have to do my laundry.

Get your workout by using a washboard (no, not a bodybuilder's stomach). Scrub your clothes for 20 minutes and there you have a workout. It will be a unique cardiovascular exercise, using your arms instead of your legs. For additional exercise, hang your clothes on a line.

You can also get out and exercise while your clothes are in a washer or dryer. For example, warm up during the washer's filling phase, have the bulk workout time during the cleaning, and cool down while your clothes spin. You know that you do not have to watch your clothes wash and dry if you are cleaning them at home. It is a little tough, though, at a laundromat, because someone could steal your clothes while you are gone. Who wants to steal wet clothes, though? Exercise during the washing phase.

 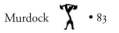

32

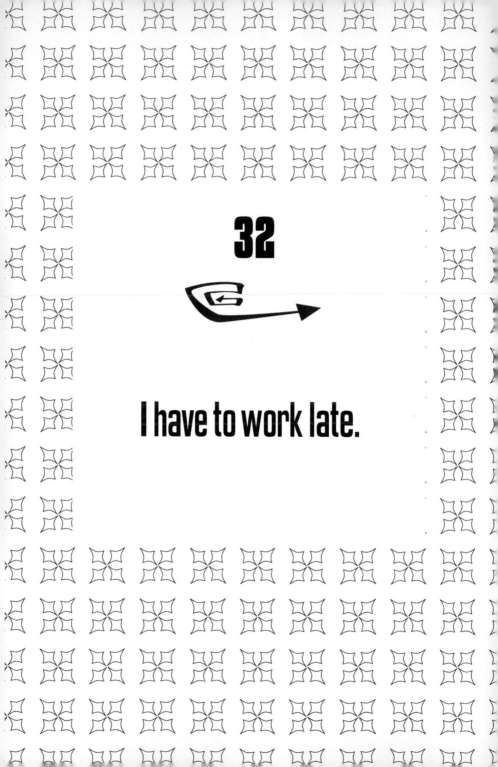

I have to work late.

If you have to work late, you should have an additional break coming to you. Take time away to exercise and then go back and finish working. Even if you take just 15 minutes to go for a walk, it will be great. You probably will be more alert, less stressed, and faster at problem solving than if you had not exercised. I find that my creativity and logic is enhanced by exercise.

Often, people have meetings after work. Suggest that the employees go for a walk, while discussing the topic at hand. Or ask if the meeting can start 20 minutes after the end of the shift to allow time to exercise.

Even if it is dark outside when you get home, you can still exercise outdoors. Light-colored clothes, a reflective vest, and flashlight are necessary to make sure that you are seen by cars. Use a bike light if you decide to ride. Women, especially, take a buddy with you.

Entrepreneurs and self-employed people, you can take a break whenever you want. Be sure to make time for exercise. Do not let work become more important than your health. After all, your career will be short if you are sick. Take care of yourself now, and you will have more time to put into your career. Lastly, your healthy lifestyle habits can influence your employee's habits. When employees are healthy, you will pay less workman's compensation and lower health insurance premiums.

 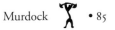

33

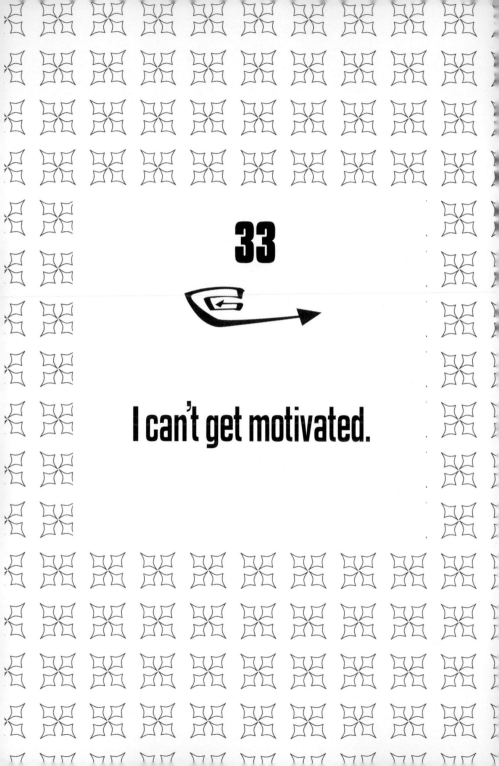

I can't get motivated.

See excuse number 29. Not being able to get psyched-up for exercise is due to lack of motivation.

Make goals for yourself and plan a reward—something that you really like such as clothes, movie, cultural event, or travel—each time you reach a goal. Never use food as a reward or punishment. That is not why we eat; food is nourishment. Make sure that your long- and short-term goals are realistic, so that they are attainable.

Choose an exercise partner or join an exercise group or club. You can motivate each other not only to meet for exercise, but also to try your best. If there is a day when you can't get motivated call up an exercise buddy and ask for support.

 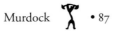

34

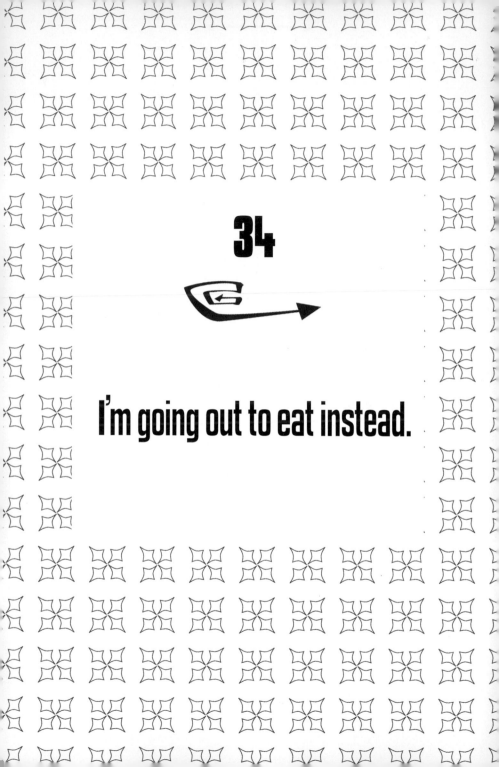

I'm going out to eat instead.

Yes, I can hear what you are thinking: "Well, I *have* to eat." This is true, but you also *have* to exercise. Do your workout as planned, then go out to eat. Your body will metabolize the food better if you exercise first, and will be less likely to store the food as fat. Leading a healthy lifestyle means having a balance between nutrition and exercise. They are of equal importance.

Walk or bike to the restaurant. Call ahead to see if there are bike racks near your destination. If you have someone going with you, have him meet you at your house. You both can reap the benefits of a pre-meal jaunt. Otherwise, walk to meet your friends at the restaurant, and then ask for a ride home after the meal.

Ask if the meeting time can be a little bit later, even just 30 minutes. That will give you plenty of time to exercise before dinner.

This excuse is the perfect opportunity to go to that restaurant that always has a 45-minute wait on Friday nights. After putting your name on the waiting list, walk around the area for 30 minutes. By the time you come back, your table will be almost ready. You will not only be healthier, but less stressed than those who sat and waited the whole time for their name to be called.

Another bonus, especially if you are trying to lose body fat, is that exercise can suppress your appetite. Workout right before eating and you will probably eat moderately. Forget about buffets if you are a compulsive overeater or have any trouble at all controlling your portions.

 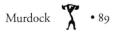

35

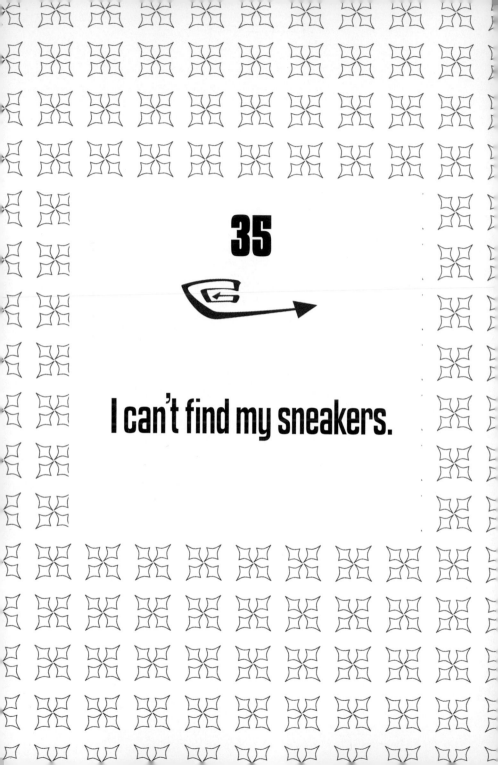

I can't find my sneakers.

Did you check the closet? Did you check your gym bag or locker? Did you check your car? Did you check your honey's home? Did you check your dog's mouth? Did you check your roommate's feet? If you answered yes to all of these but still could not find them, it is time to pick a different mode of exercise.

Swimming is a great mode for which you do not need any special shoes. Even if you cannot swim, you can exercise in the shallow end, doing shallow-water walking or running.

There are exercise tools called AquaJoggers™, which are worn around the waist to keep you afloat. They are great for performing deep-water running, walking, and strength training in a pool's deep end. Runners should seriously consider intermittently using the pool to help prevent overuse injuries like shin splints, stress fractures (a bone break caused by a sudden force at the point of muscular attachment), and Achilles' tendonitis (inflammation of the tissue that connects the calf muscles to the heel bone).

If you do not know how to swim, now is a great time to learn. You never know when you might need swimming skills to survive or to save someone else's life. Call your local YMCA for more information.

Other choices for exercise when you cannot find your special shoes are bicycling, weight lifting, stationary rowing, and stair climbing. Never give up on getting your exercise for the day. You can always find a different mode until your sneakers show up.

Do not search so hard that you get stressed. You are looking for your sneakers to improve your health, not to elevate your blood pressure.

 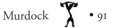

36

I have car trouble.

This is the perfect opportunity to exercise. I had a 1969 VW Bug for six and a half years, during which time I exercised a lot. Every time it broke down, I had to ride my bike, skate, or walk to work, school, and stores. Also, I biked to the auto shop when I needed to consult with the mechanic.

Have you ever taken your car in to get it checked and were told it would only take a few minutes? Well, you might as well tell them that you would return in a few minutes. Go for a walk while you are waiting for a diagnosis, then return to the auto shop. If you consent to having the work done, go out for another walk. It will help you cool down and stay calm about your car being broken and about how much it will cost to get it fixed.

Have you ever had your car stall in the street—worse yet, the middle of an intersection? Pushing a car is great exercise, especially when you do not have any help. Once when I was out skating I saw someone stall in the middle of the intersection. I pushed his car across the street and next to a curb. What a workout!

If you do not have any way of getting to your usual workout area, just exercise in or around your home. Walk, bike, or skate outside or dance indoors to your favorite music. This is also a great time to accomplish yardwork or housecleaning. ACSM (4) includes those chores as two of several modes of exercise that we should do five times a week for 30 minutes each.

Keep a pair of sneakers in your car. You never know when you are going to get stuck and need to walk for help, or have some free time to exercise.

37

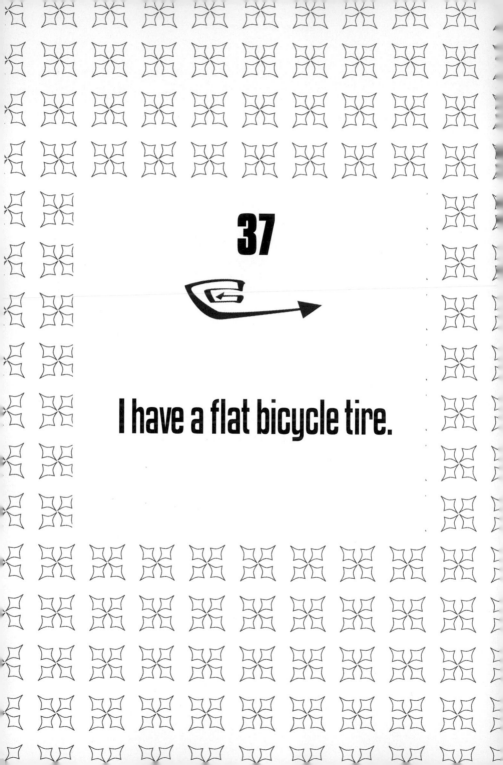

I have a flat bicycle tire.

My friend, Gina, and I have seen so many people walking their broken bikes that now we say, "Look! That guy is taking his bike for a walk." You will be in for more exercise than you had planned if you get a flat tire while out riding, and do not have a tire repair kit. It's even worse if you are out mountain biking and need to walk your bike back over rugged terrain, or stay and fix it on uneven ground. Be prepared. Bicycle shops sell handy cases (which look like miniature fanny packs) that attach to a seat and can hold a phone and a tire repair kit (also available at bicycle stores).

When you notice your flat tire before you start riding, just walk it down to the bicycle shop, walk around while it's being fixed, and then go for your ride. If you are out of time after the bike has been fixed, that is OK. At least you did do some exercising, which is better than staying home and being stressed about your bike.

For those of you do-it-yourselfers who have little free time, walk for a few minutes, reserving some time to fix your tire. You will have had at least *some* exercise and a clearer, calmer mind to take care of your bike.

38

I have to take my child to ___.

Walk your child to the destination, and then walk home. You can drive when you need to pick up your child.

Encourage the family to bicycle to destinations. If you have a child, get an extra seat for your bike or have him ride his own bike. Make sure your child wears a helmet, as required by many state laws.

My mom used to drive me everywhere when I was younger, since we lived in a city where only the schools were within walking distances. She drove me to where I wanted to go, drove home, picked me up later, and then drove home, again. Sometimes, she just sat in the car and waited for me. Make good use of your time by exercising while you wait for your child at the doctor or dentist's office, movie theatre, pizza parlor, mall, or sport's practice. You can walk around that area or drive to your gym for a workout. Try planning your child's appointment around your favorite exercise class, so that you accomplish two things at once.

Teach your children healthy habits. Have your children walk or bike to their destinations whenever feasible. Don't worry if they complain, they will thank you later. Do not teach them that if they complain enough, they can get out of exercising. You do not want them growing up and giving me more book material. Teach the route to school, by walking with your child, and soon he will be able to do it on his own. If it is a bad neighborhood, walk with your child each way, each day, and get a lot of exercise!

The less driving you do, the more your child will benefit from exercising and the more time you will have for your own workouts.

 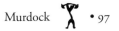

39

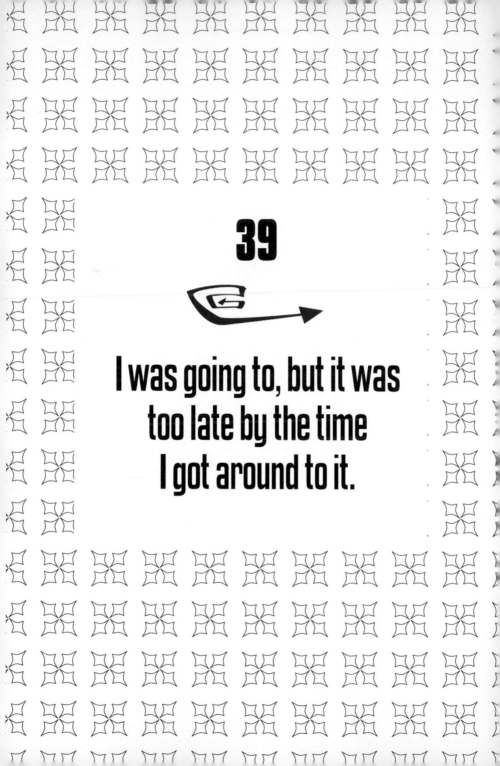

I was going to, but it was too late by the time I got around to it.

For those of you who use this excuse a lot, there are two things you can do: 1) make an appointment for yourself to exercise, and/or 2) exercise first thing in the morning. Make the appointment like you would for anything else that requires a commitment to someone else. The only difference is that this time it would be a commitment to you. If you have an appointment book, write "Exercise" at a given time—in ink—and do not cancel or reschedule. Try to make the appointment for the same time each day. For example, every Tuesday and Thursday at 3 p.m. and every Monday, Wednesday, and Friday at 2 p.m. Keep the appointment like you would for anything else that is important to you and exercise will become habitual. Do not let anything take precedence over it. The second option of getting around this excuse is exercising first thing in the morning. Get up, eat, visit the bathroom, get dressed, and exercise. In that order? Yes. It is a good idea to eat first, so that you leave some time for your food to digest and so that you do not exercise on an empty stomach. Eating first gives your body a chance to wake up and avoid having exercise be such a shock. What is the best thing to eat before exercising? What you normally eat. You do not need to eat something special before exercising, but if you normally have eggs and bacon every morning, you probably need to change your whole diet, anyway. Also pertaining to order, it is highly recommended that you dress before you go out, unless you want people to see you in your pajamas or unless you where spandex to bed.

I am not quick to recommend getting up earlier to fit exercise into your schedule. Awaking at a different time (earlier or later) than normal, can make you very tired, by throwing off your **circadian rhythm** (biological clock). Unless you really want to commit to getting up five or more times a week earlier than usual and changing your rhythm, I do not recommend it. The success rate for people trying to get up earlier than usual to exercise is low. Instead, I recommend exercising first thing in the morning, after rising at your usual time, and starting and ending your workday later.

Another option if you find yourself at the end of the day saying you never got around to exercising is doing it right then and there. Quit talking and go to the gym (most of which are open late), dance around to your favorite music, bike (wearing light or reflective clothing and using a bike light), or walk (be sure you are with a buddy, if you're female). Even if you exercise for 20 minutes, it will be beneficial and probably help you sleep well.

 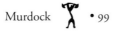

40

I have to clean the house.

This is not a bad excuse, actually. You can get a lot of exercise by cleaning, especially if you have not cleaned in a while or you have a big home. Turn on some music and make it fun! OK. I cannot believe I just said that—cleaning is never fun for me no matter what I am playing, but heavy metal music helps. Anyway, if you spend your workout time cleaning, you might as well burn a lot of Calories while you are at it and accomplish two things at once.

You can also spend less time on housework by getting someone to help you, and then you can exercise together afterward. Later, take your helper for a healthy meal to thank her.

 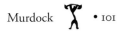

41

I have to catch up
on my reading.

Unless, of course, your reading includes this book, it is not a valid excuse. Take your reading to the gym. You will not have any problem getting it done, since most cardiovascular equipment (stationary bike, treadmill, stairclimber) has a built-in reading rack or one that can be placed on a machine's control panel. You can also read in between strength training sets while you are resting. Don't read during the set, because you need to concentrate on the muscles you are working. It has been proven that there is more stimulation at the muscle site when you are thinking about it. If you do not know which muscles you are working, be sure to ask a trainer. Most strength training equipment made these days have diagrams of the muscles being worked. Do not try to read during an aerobics class, either—you might trip and fall.

If you have cardiovascular equipment at home, invest in a reading rack. It can be found at a sporting goods store or wherever you bought your equipment.

When I was in school, I used to save time by studying for a test while walking outside, flashcards in hand. It worked out well, because walking cleared my head and helped me to concentrate on my studies.

Nowadays to catch up on my reading, I bring a magazine or book with me wherever I go. Often I arrive early to my appointments, so I sit in the car and read for a few minutes. The few minutes here and there add up quickly and before I know it I have all of my reading done. Also, it seems there are places where I must always wait, like the car wash, the doctor's office, or the post office. At each place I wait patiently, knowing that I am wisely spending my time reading. It helps to prevent certain situations from being perceived as stressful, too.

 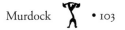

42

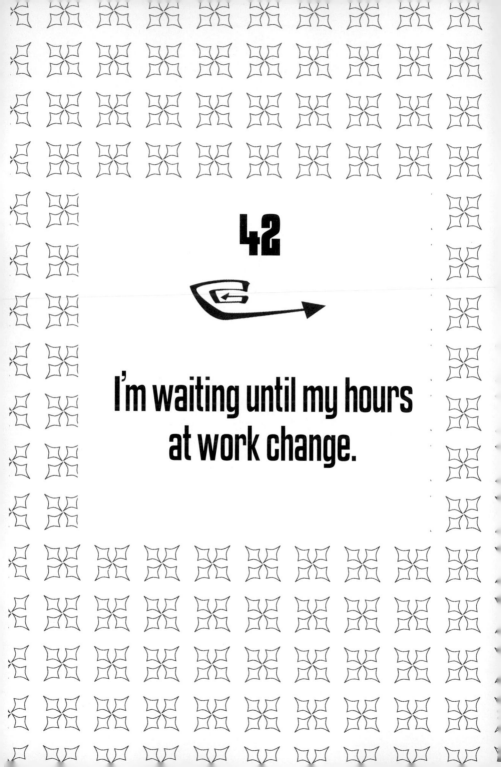

I'm waiting until my hours at work change.

If you are like most people, you are going to have changes all of the time. When we know that a change is about to occur or is in the process of occurring, we cannot stop everything else we are doing until the change is established. We need to use our time management skills to accommodate all of our responsibilities, like exercising.

No matter what work hours, activities, other responsibilities, or crises you have, you need to make time for exercise. People want to make duties as convenient as possible, especially the ones they do not enjoy, including exercise. Convenience is not always possible, though, so the more important tasks become a priority. Make exercise one of your more (if not most) important tasks. Make time now to exercise and make time when your schedule changes.

If you know what your new hours will be, start planning when you will exercise. Write it in your planner, on your calendar, or on a piece of paper and try to keep the time consistent so it will become a habit.

Start an exercise program now or comply with a pre-existing one and stay healthy (or become healthier) through your changes.

 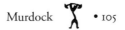

43

I forgot my gym clothes.

Workout naked!* Have you seen T-shirts that say "ski naked" or "surf naked"? What about one that says "workout naked"?

Seriously. You were planning on going to the gym straight from work, but forgot your gym clothes. You could stop at a store and get that exercise outfit you have always wanted; go home and then to the gym; exercise at or around home; or even buy or borrow clothes from the gym.

After your workout, develop a system so that you remember your gym clothes. Keep your gym clothes in your car until they require washing. If you wash your clothes after every workout or like to wear a different outfit each day, keep a back-up outfit in the car. It will always be there for you to use in case you forget your gym clothes. Prepare your clothes before you go to bed and put them by the front door, in your car, or under your car keys. For those of you who spend five minutes in the morning looking for the keys, the last idea is not a good one for you, obviously. Otherwise, you might need a "Clapper" for your clothes, too.

*Do not try this. It is a joke.

 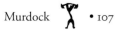

44

My dog ate my exercise log.

To prevent losing your workout plan, write it on the computer.

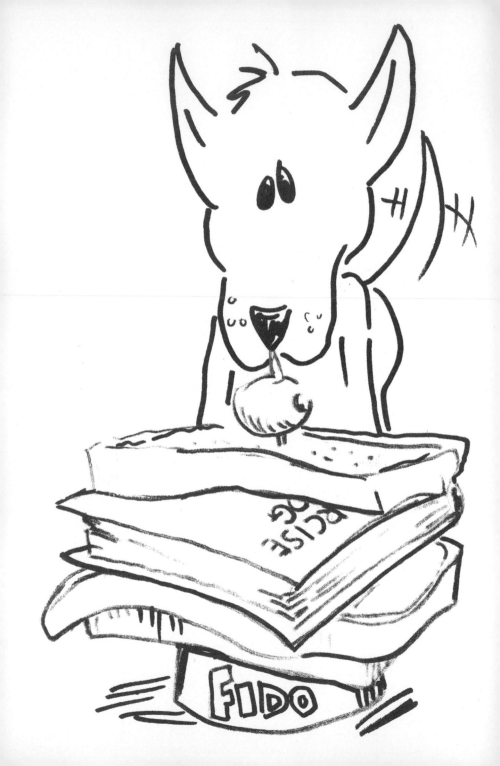

Time to get out the **activated charcoal** or **Ipecac Syrup**^{TM}.* Maybe even try the doggy **Heimlich Maneuver**.*

Do your best to remember the exercises. Otherwise call your trainer, if that is who made the workout, and write the exercises on a note pad. Remember to ask the trainer to bring a new card to your next session. If you belong to a gym and your trainer cannot be reached, ask another trainer to teach you some exercises for the day. If you can't remember your exercises or reach your trainer, go for a walk.

To prevent losing your workout plan, write it on the computer. You can print a new copy whenever you need it.

*Do not try this. It is a joke.

 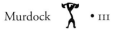

45

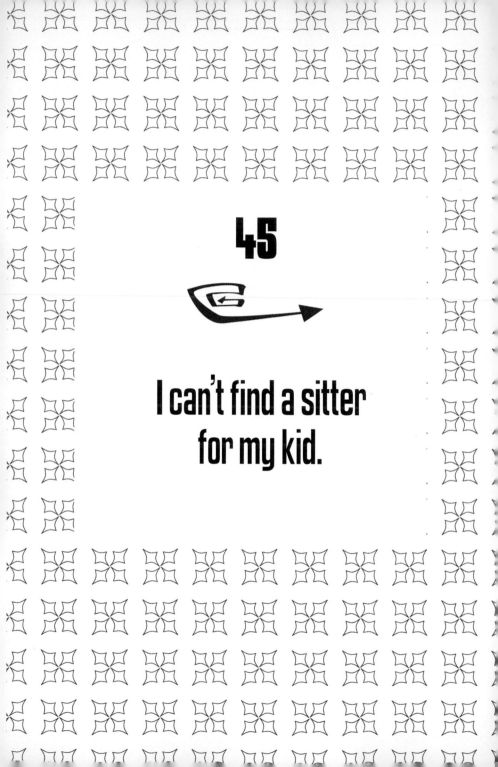

I can't find a sitter for my kid.

Take your kid to the gym with you. A lot of gyms offer childcare. If your gym does not, suggest that they do and get your parent friends at the gym to do the same. With enough demand, the gym might offer the additional service.

Do not spend too much time trying to find a sitter. You will just get stressed during which time you can be exercising. Take your child out for a walk or to the playground where you can climb up and down the ladders, go across the monkey bars, play on a rope, and swing. Believe me, it will feel like more of a workout than your usual routine. I speak from experience and so can my clients. It is tough—especially, if you have not played in years. Be careful when trying what you did as a kid. You may break something or be extremely sore later.

 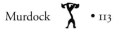

46

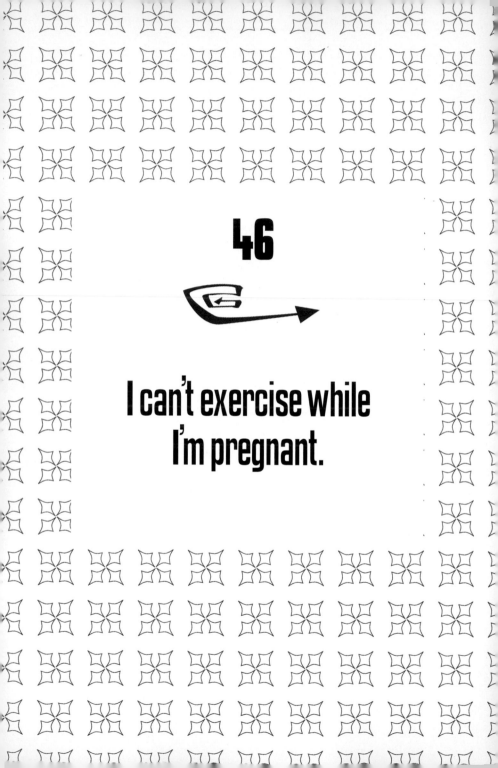

I can't exercise while I'm pregnant.

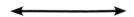

One can and should exercise while pregnant because of the benefits. Consult your obstetrician, first. "Benefits of a properly designed **prenatal** exercise program include: improved aerobic and muscular fitness, facilitat(ed) . . . recovery from labor, enhanced maternal psychological well-being, and establish(ed,) . . . permanent healthy lifestyle habits" (4). The ability to maintain proper posture and reduce the frequency and intensity of back pain; weight control; improvement in digestion; reduction in constipation; energy improvement; and a decrease in chance of "**postpartum** belly" are other benefits (4).

When one exercises during pregnancy, guidelines should be followed closely (2):

1. Mild to moderate exercise at least three times per week.
2. To avoid excessive reduction in **fetal** blood flow, avoid: a) the supine (on your back) position after the first **trimester**; b) vigorous exercise; c) and prolonged periods of motionless standing.
3. Stop exercising when fatigued—do not wait until exhausted.
4. Weight-bearing exercises are fine, but non-weight-bearing exercises reduce the chance for injury.
5. As gestation (pregnancy) progresses, especially after the second trimester, balance exercises should be avoided. Due to the mother's center of gravity changing, it is more likely she could fall when trying to balance.
6. Avoid exercises with the potential for even mild abdominal trauma.
7. Ensure adequate diet.
8. Stay well hydrated and cool.
9. Resume exercise gradually after birth, according to physical capability.

Be sure to stop exercising, though, if any of the following occur (and seek medical advice) (48):

1. Any "gush" of fluid or bloody discharge from the **vagina**.
2. Sudden swelling of face, hands, or ankles.
3. Persistent, severe headache, dizziness, faintness, and/or visual disturbances.
4. Blood pressure or pulse rate that stays elevated after exercise.
5. Excessive fatigue, chest pains, and/or **palpitations**.
6. Persistent contractions (> six to eight/hour) that may suggest onset of premature labor.
7. Unexplained abdominal pain.
8. Insufficient weight gain [< 1.0 kg/month (< 2.2 pounds/month)] during the last two trimesters). Severe **anemia**, phlebitis (inflammation of the veins), significant infection, or other significant medical problems, are other reasons to discontinue an exercise program.

Lastly, one may not even be able to start exercising if certain conditions exist. They include pregnancy-induced hypertension, pre-term rupture of membrane, pre-term labor during the prior or current pregnancy, incompetent **cervix**, persistent second to third trimester bleeding, and/or **intrauterine** growth retardation (2).

 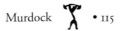

47

I broke a nail and need
to go get it fixed.

Have an emergency nail repair kit at home. This way your nail can look decent, and you won't miss your workout. You can see your manicurist at a more convenient time. Do not give up exercise for a nail. The inside of your body is much more important than the outside.

Find ways to prevent a nail brake from happening in the first place. Think about using a better manicurist, higher quality nails, or go al naturale (no fake nails—my favorite).

Suggest that your manicurist get a recumbent bike in her salon. Then you could exercise and get your nail fixed at once and save time!

 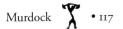

48

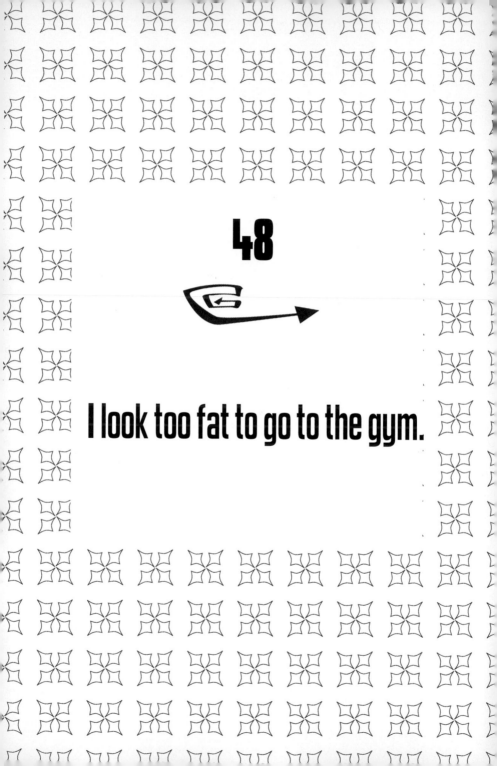

I look too fat to go to the gym.

If you are too self-conscious to be seen in a gym, exercise outdoors or at home. That is one reason why home gyms are so popular—the public will not see you. Also, you do not have to wear a thong leotard or even brush your hair. Now, if exercising at home is absolutely out of the question, swallow your pride and get out and walk. Whatever it takes, do it, even if that means dressing incognito with a trench coat and nun's hat in the middle of summer. Just go! If you think you do not have enough self-confidence to get outside and exercise, probably nothing will change that except for one thing. Exercise! Not only will the physiological effects of exercise make you feel better, but also just doing it can raise your self-esteem (39).

Remember the importance and reasons why you would go to the gym in the first place. It is not to be accepted by others, but by yourself and to improve your health. Exercising around others (at a gym), especially in a class, can motivate you to return consistently for your workouts. If you see your committed acquaintances coming to class (like it or not) and benefiting from exercise, you will do the same. Having gym friends will create a support system that is sure to give you a boost each time you go. Also, a good gym will have reputable trainers than can design a personalized workout for you, including teaching you safe techniques.

49

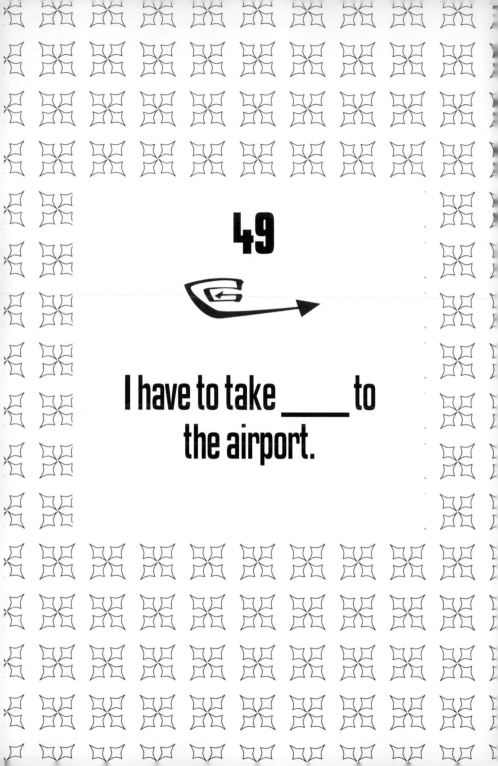

I have to take ____ to the airport.

What a perfect place to exercise, especially if the airport is Chicago's O'Hare. Walking from one gate to another, or gate to baggage claim, is a workout in itself. Add a suitcase or two and you are burning serious Calories.

When taking people (or yourself) to the airport, plan to park and walk them to the security area. This way you will not lose a day of exercise. Go up stairs instead of elevators or escalators. If there are no stairs, walk or run up the escalators. Avoid the moving walkways—walk on the carpet. Allow enough time to get around the airport, so you will not think that you need the walkways. When there is a flight delay or you arrive extra early to the airport, use the time to get more exercise instead of sitting. Walk around the airport some more, locking up your bags if needed. If there are no lockers, rent a cart or take turns with a friend watching the bags.

 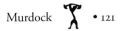

50

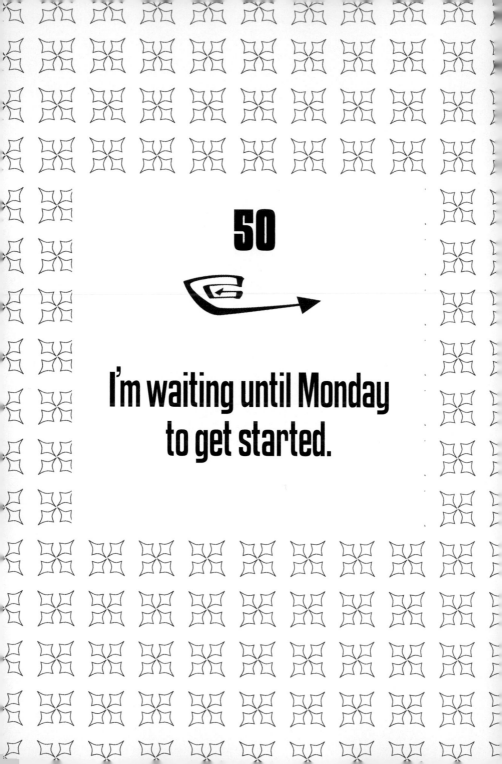

I'm waiting until Monday to get started.

Why wait to reap the benefits of exercise? Feel well today—be proud of yourself today! The farther away Monday is, the more difficult it will be to start and the longer it will take you to reach your exercise goal.

Do you know what your exercise goals are? Take some time to think about them and write them down. Be realistic, though. If you are a female built short and stout, do not make looking like Christie Brinkley your goal. If you are a male built tall and thin, do not expect to look like Arnold Schwarzennegger. Having goals is motivating, since it is exciting to think how much better we can look and feel.

Go out and get some exercise today. Just do something, even if it is for only five minutes. This will be your start of a life-long commitment to exercise, and the start of a habit. Why not go right now? Put this book down and exercise now, whether it is walking, going up and down your stairs, or shooting some hoops. You can resume your reading when you get back. Go!

 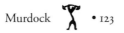

51

I'm waiting until the
first of the year.

My response to this is not too different from the one above, except now I must assume that the waiting time is long. Think about all of the New Year's resolutions you have made in the past. What percentage of those were you able to keep throughout the year? They usually do not stick because they are made for the wrong reason. Be unique and start making positive changes today. Exercise! Start now.

The longer you wait the more you will lose, thanks to the aging process. For example, it is normal to have a decline in $\dot{V}O_2$ max (aerobic power), but through exercise we can control how much. "In older endurance competitors, a decrease of about 8 ml/kg/min of VO_2 max occurred between 35 and 65 years of age, compared to a steady decline in the average person of 4-5 ml/kg/min *per decade* from age 25 to 65 (27). The rate of decline of VO_2 max is therefore 33-45% slower in endurance-trained competitors compared to the average population" (7). Oxygen consumption is directly related to metabolism. The more oxygen a cell is consuming, the more Calories it is burning, and therefore the higher the metabolism.

Also related to metabolism is the amount of muscle mass one has. Muscle consumes more Calories than fat does to sustain itself. Therefore, the more muscle you have the higher your metabolism. As we age, we lose muscle mass no matter what, but through exercise—especially strength training—we can gain muscle mass now (up to our potential) then sustain as much as possible as we age. Remember that as metabolism slows, the likelihood to gain fat increases.

Phillips and Cureton performed a study on six middle-aged subjects. The experiment was held at the University of Illinois, where the subjects were trained for eight weeks, de-trained for eight weeks, and re-trained for eight weeks. During the first eight weeks, the subjects gradually progressed from 30 minutes of calisthenics, 30 minutes of cross-country running, and then 30 minutes of handball. After the initial eight weeks, the program was discontinued and the men returned to a sedentary life, performing the usual minimal activities of life. Then, the third eight-week session consisted of a program somewhat longer and harder than what they had followed the first eight weeks. Throughout the 24 weeks, the men were able to eat whatever they wanted.

Phillips and Cureton took measurements once each month on the subjects. They found that there were improvements during the first few weeks, but the greater improvements were in the last eight weeks. On average, the subjects' **basal metabolic rate** (BMR) increased 23%, suggesting an increase in muscle mass (8).

Other effects of aging that we can control include loss of flexibility and bone, and slow reaction time. An effective exercise program can improve all of these, so get started! Go!

 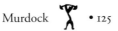

52

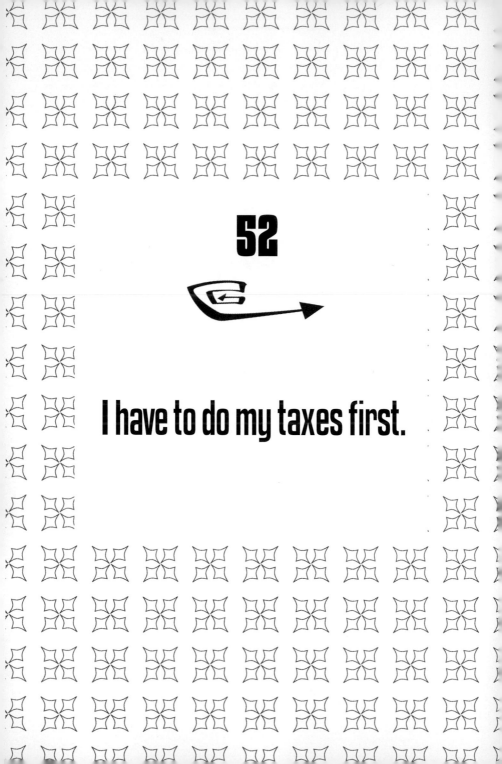

I have to do my taxes first.

Exercise first. You will probably have a clearer head and be less stressed, a combination that could help prevent mistakes. If it is 11 p.m. on April 14th, do your taxes first. Having the IRS after you is worse than not exercising. After you do your taxes and exercise, sign up for a class to cure another problem—procrastination. Plan your time wisely, so that you will not have to use this excuse, even if it is not April 14th.

Doing your own taxes can take a long time even if you know what you are doing. Take frequent exercise breaks (10 minutes will do) to separate the monotony. Seriously think about hiring a certified public accountant (CPA), because it will save you money. All of the time that you spend doing taxes yourself is worth more than a CPA would charge. You will have more time left over to exercise!!

If you have access to a stationary machine like a bike, you can exercise while you read over paper work, including files. Invite your CPA to the gym, or better yet your home (if you have equipment at home), where you can field questions while exercising. Do not try to do this while strength training, because you need to concentrate on form (not the tax type), the muscles being worked, and not dropping free weights. If your CPA does not make housecalls, suggest that he get a treadmill or bike in his office. It would be a great way to keep his clients calm and of course healthy. The healthier his clients, the longer they will live, and the longer they have to pay taxes.

 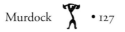

53

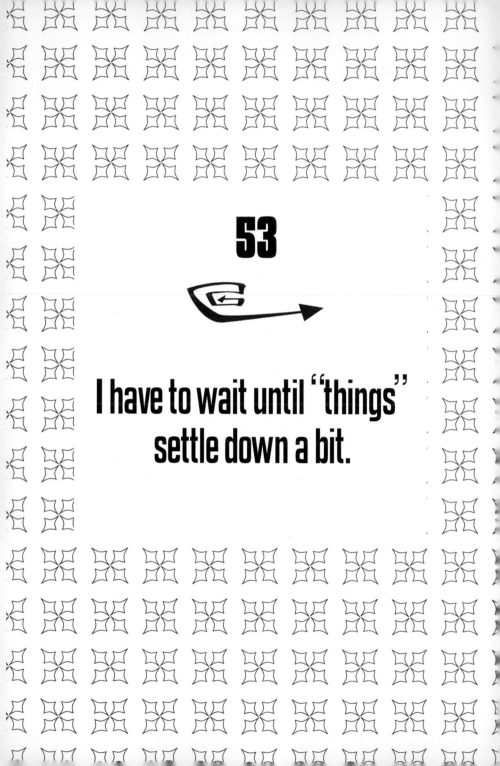

I have to wait until "things" settle down a bit.

See numbers 3 and 24, also.

If you are like a lot of people, your life will never settle down. That is what makes life so exciting. There is always something to do. The challenge is to enumerate each task according to importance, such as having exercise at the top of the list and cleaning at the bottom.

No, you do not have to wait until things settle down a bit. How you lead your life is entirely up to you. You control your own outcome and perception of life's events.

Dr. Michael Mantell once said:

"RULE NO. 1: DON'T SWEAT THE SMALL STUFF. RULE NO. 2.: IT'S ALL SMALL STUFF."

 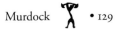

54

I'm waiting for the weather to get nicer.

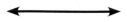

Whatever is nicer to you is probably a range of a few degrees like 75° to 80° F. You cannot always count on that weather, so you will need to find a way to stay warmer or cooler depending on the temperature. If you do wait, it may be a long time. Remember, the longer you wait for the temperature to change, the longer it will take you to reach your goal. You may even store additional fat, which means you will need additional exercise. What if in the next hour the weather does get nicer. Will you really exercise then?

If you are one who always uses the weather as an excuse, you might be a candidate for home exercise. Think about how much your home and budget allow for exercise equipment. You do not even have to get something fancy from the local sporting goods store; look in the newspaper's classified ads, swap meets, or garage sales for used equipment. You might find an exercise bicycle or free weights.

 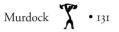

55

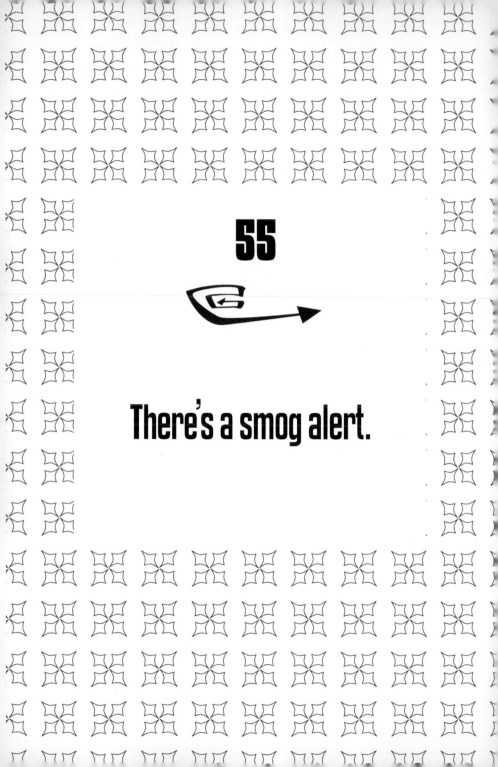

There's a smog alert.

This, actually, is a decent excuse, but not good enough. During smog alert, use an indoor pool, gym, or your home to exercise. It is all right if you do not complete your usual workout, since you will still be in the habit of doing some exercise.

During smog alert, you should not exercise outdoors. "Carbon monoxide (CO), the most common air pollutant, can substantially inhibit athletic performance," says research physiologist Peter Frykman of the U. S. Army Research Institute of Environmental Medicine in Natick, MA. "It prevents blood from carrying the normal concentration of oxygen to muscles, which in turn forces the heart to pump more blood to meet the demands of exercise" (10).

Cities such as Denver, Los Angeles, New York, and Phoenix can have over 100 parts per million (ppm) of CO (safe is 35 ppm or less) during rush hour. Exercising in this level for 30 minutes can be like smoking a half-pack to a full-pack of cigarettes.

Ozone, a colorless gas created by the action of ultraviolet light on automotive emissions, is a major component of smog. Ozone can cause respiratory problems in otherwise healthy people. If you have chest tightness, eye irritation, coughing, or shortness of breath after exercising on a smoggy day, it is probably from the ozone.

If unsure about the smog level in your area, check the Pollutant Standard Index (PSI) level before exercising outdoors to make sure it is below 100 ppm. Try exercising in the morning, avoiding busy roadways, and steering clear of secondhand cigarette smoke before and after exercise. Better yet, always avoid secondhand cigarette smoke. If you smoke, you have more things to worry about than smog. Anytime you have trouble breathing, stop exercising (10).

 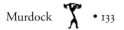

56

I drove by the gym, but I couldn't get myself to stop.

Did you try using the brakes? If that does not work, try using the emergency brake.* If that doesn't work either, you can shut off the engine and coast to the gym parking lot.*

Stay in the habit of going to the gym on the days that you planned. The more exercise days you miss the harder it will be to "stop." Think about the guilt that you will have if you do not go. You will feel worse from it than if you had not planned on going at all.

Plan on meeting someone there. It will be much harder to break the commitment to someone else than to yourself. Better yet, find someone at work to go with you—someone who will make sure you will stop at the gym. Remember: NO MORE DRIVE-BYS.

*Do not try this. It is a joke.

 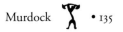

57

My spouse told me I had to come right home after work, so I couldn't go to the gym.

If you told your spouse you were planning on going to the bar after work, she might tell you that you "had to come right home." But it would not be right for her to tell you this if you were planning to exercise. Tell her how important it is for you to exercise. Maybe only an exercising spouse would understand.

Try to get a non-exercising spouse to workout with you. Gyms often offer special deals if spouses sign up together. Plan to go to the gym together, motivate each other, and commit to lifelong fitness.

Trying to keep the peace in a household is definitely an important matter. If you must go home right from work, make a point to exercise at or around home, before dinner perhaps. Pick up dinner on the way home so that you will not be expected to cook or clean up, leaving more time to exercise. If your spouse has an important matter to discuss, talk while walking. You both may feel more relaxed, and you'll be in neutral territory.

 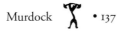

58

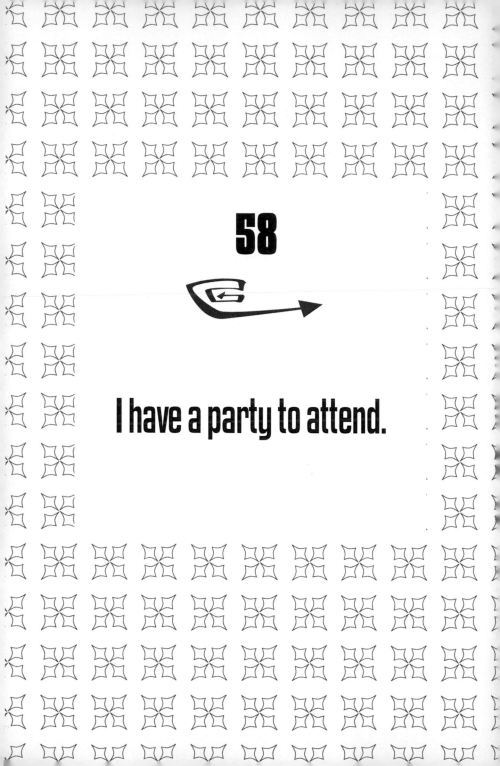

I have a party to attend.

You can skip your usual workout, if you know the party will have an activity involving exercise.

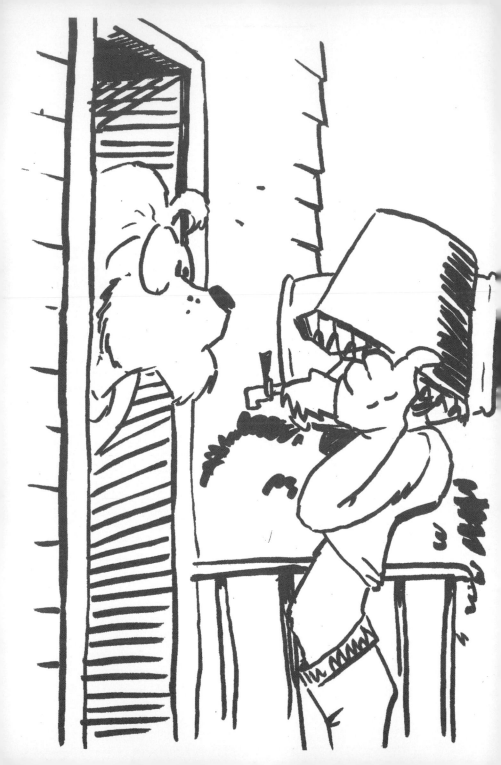

If the party has dancing, limbo, or swimming, this is an acceptable excuse. You can skip your usual workout, if you know the party will have an activity involving exercise. Do not skip a strength training workout, though, because it is too easy for the muscles to forget how they were stressed. At least complete one set [group of repetitions (movements)] of each exercise, thereby maintaining the muscle strength, mass, **tonicity**, and endurance you worked so hard to achieve. Waiting too long (more than five days) between strength training sessions will cause regression.

Promote exercise and overall wellness by having exercise-related activities at your own parties. You want your friends to be around and healthy for a long time, right? Get them together for a softball game, pool party (you can play pool volleyball), a beach or lake party, or a skating party. Encourage friends to play Smashball™, volleyball, Frisbee, or football at the beach or lake.

When having your own party, promote wellness by offering non-alcoholic beverages and healthier snacks like carrot and celery sticks. Encourage healthy dishes and drinks for potlucks, too. By eliminating alcohol from a party, you will be able to sleep well, knowing that all of your friends made it home without causing a drunk-driving collision.

 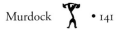

59

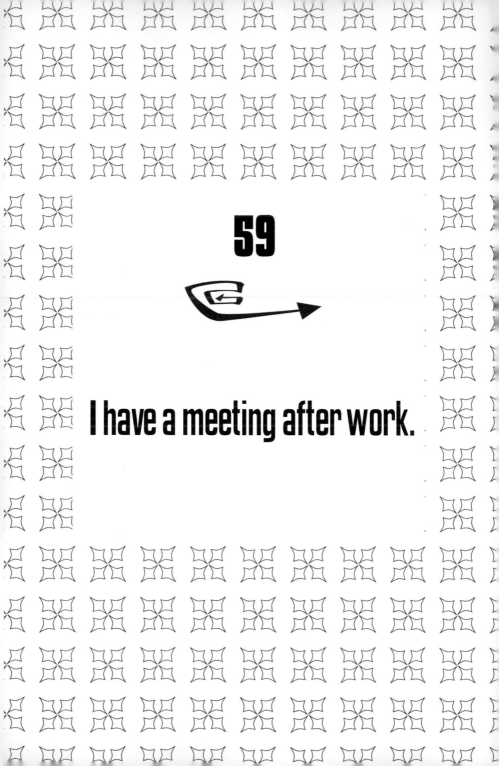

I have a meeting after work.

That is OK. Exercise before work or at lunchtime. Exercise so that you can stay on your workout schedule. You do not even have to go to the gym or your usual spot. You do not even have to change your clothes. Just go for a walk near where you work—even for just 15 minutes. It is helpful, though, to wear comfortable footwear such as walking, running, or cross-training shoes.

Encourage the boss to hold a meeting outside—a walk and talk. Everyone can walk, while discussing current issues. Walk for just part of the meeting, when you know you will not need a visual aid like an overhead projector. Although, most overheads have wheels—take it with you.* Some meetings can be pretty stressful (and boring) and walking can not only help keep people relaxed, but also awake.

If you do not get to workout before or during the meeting, exercise afterward. Exercising will probably make you feel better after a long meeting and prevent you from feeling guilty about not exercising.

*Do not try this. It is a joke.

 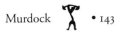

60

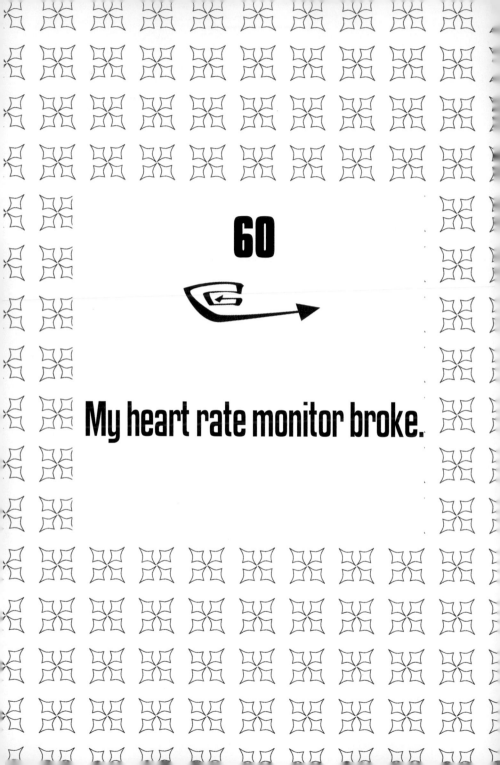

My heart rate monitor broke.

Take your heart rate manually. The best two places for measuring your pulse are your carotid artery (side of neck) and wrist (front/thumb side of forearm). Use your second and third fingers (pointer and longest fingers) to feel your pulse. When using the carotid artery, press gently so that you do not cut off the blood flow to your brain.

Let us say that you have an analog clock and want to start measuring your pulse when the second hand gets to the twelve. To start, count "zero" in your head, the next beat you feel is "one" and so on. Measure your pulse for ten seconds and multiply the number of beats by six. The product will be beats per minute. If you counted 20 beats in the 10 seconds, your heart rate is 120 beats per minute [20 (beats) x 6 = 120 beats per minute].

It is normal for there to be error by those who are inexperienced in measuring heart rate, so do not be discouraged if you get it wrong. That is why you have a heart rate monitor, right? Until it is fixed, you can use what is called Borg's (34) rating of perceived exertion (RPE):

0	Nothing at all
0.5	Very, very weak
1	Very, weak
2	Weak
3	Moderate
4	Somewhat strong
5	Strong
6	
7	Very strong
8	
9	
10	Very, very strong
*	Maximal

The classification for each rating describes the intensity of the workout, according to how the exerciser feels. If you are supposed to exercise at a heart rate between 125 and 135 beats per minute, decide what RPE it is for you. Then for your next workout, you can use the above scale without measuring your pulse.

 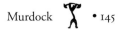

61

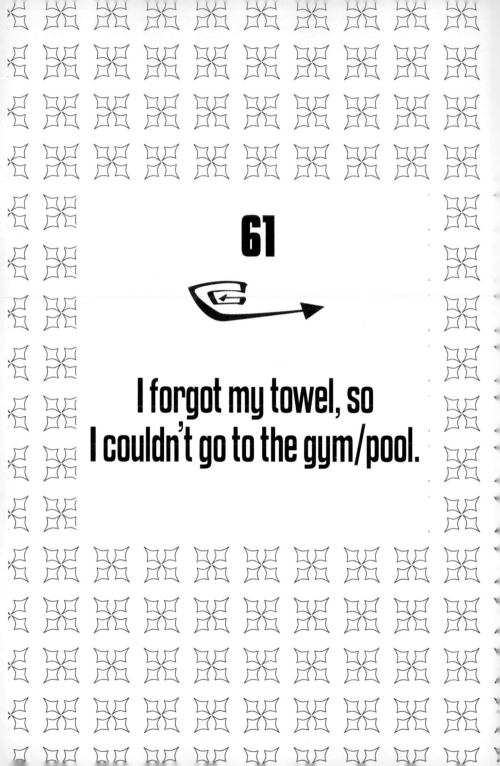

I forgot my towel, so I couldn't go to the gym/pool.

I can think of two times I was at a pool and found that I had forgotten my towel. I simply marched right into the shower area after swimming, got some paper towels, took my shower, and you can figure out the rest. It worked out well.

Most gyms offer towels at the front desk for you to borrow. As for pools, I do not know of any that lend towels, but some might sell them. Alternatively, you can buy one at a store on the way to the gym or pool.

Be spontaneous—exercise around home—by biking, walking, or skating. You will have everything you need at home, including a towel. It will be nice to do something different, and add variety to your life.

Pack wisely so that you do not forget your towel, again. Keep a spare in the car so that you will have a back up in just such an emergency.

 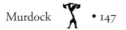

62

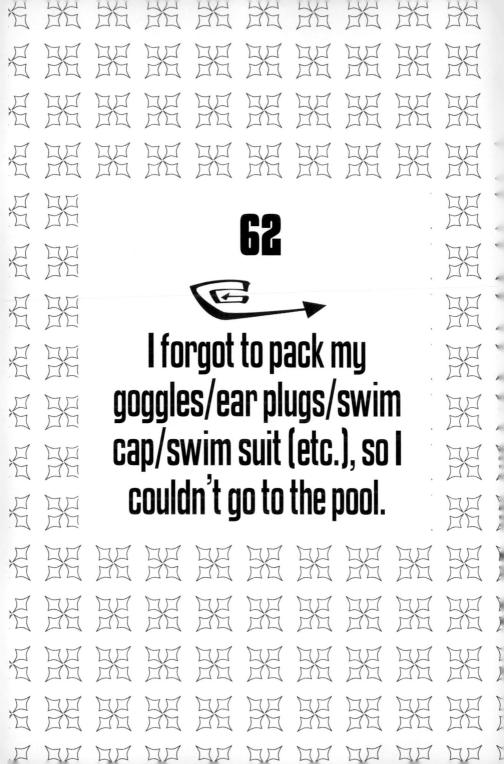

I forgot to pack my goggles/ear plugs/swim cap/swim suit (etc.), so I couldn't go to the pool.

Develop a system so that you do not forget any swimming equipment. Prepare them before you go to bed and put them by the front door, in your car, or under your car keys. Since you will need to wash your suit and towel or at least hang them to dry when you get home, make a permanent note to yourself to gather them before leaving the house.

If you forget just your goggles, ear plugs, or swim cap, try a different type of aquatic workout like shallow water walking or running or specific exercises (24).

When not prepared at all for being in the pool, do a dry-land workout. If the pool is part of a club, take an aerobics class, or use the weights or cardiovascular equipment such as a treadmill or stationary bicycle. Be sure to consult a trainer, before using the equipment for the first time, or the aerobics instructor, before taking a class for the first time. Otherwise, just go home and exercise around there. Do not let your memory lapse turn you off from exercising, or from giving less time to your workout than you had planned.

 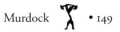

63

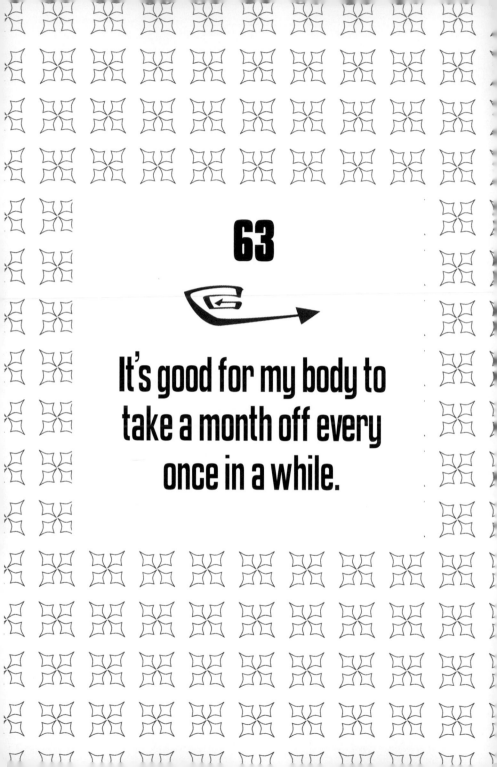

It's good for my body to take a month off every once in a while.

No, it is not. That is like saying: "It is a good idea to let myself go every once and a while." It is like yo-yo dieting, but not as bad. When one stops exercising for a prolonged period of time (e.g., a month), the muscles atrophy (get smaller) and the metabolic rate declines. If fewer Calories are burned during the day and the same Caloric intake is maintained, weight gain occurs. When you consume 3500 Calories more than you expend in one week, one pound is gained that week. We all know weight (fat) gain is not healthy. As with dieting, the more you stop and start exercising the more your body composition (percentage of body fat) fluctuates, and the harder it may be to get it down.

If you take off a month, plan on starting from scratch when you resume. No fun! Remember the last time you started an exercise program? It is hard work to increase cardiovascular and muscle endurance, muscle strength, flexibility, and tonicity. Also, there is an increased chance of injury to an untrained body, especially for someone who thinks he can pick up where he left off a month ago.

It is good to take time off occasionally, though. An exercised muscle group needs 48 hours to rest and repair after strength training, whereas cardiovascular exercise can be performed on consecutive days. For everyday exercisers, it's a good idea to take one day a week off from exercise. Seven days a week of heavy exercise will lead to injury.

Think about why you want a month off. Is it because your body feels warn out? Are you bored with your exercise routine? Do you think that you have higher priorities than your health?

64

My alarm didn't go off.

If you miss your morning workout, do it later in the day or after work.

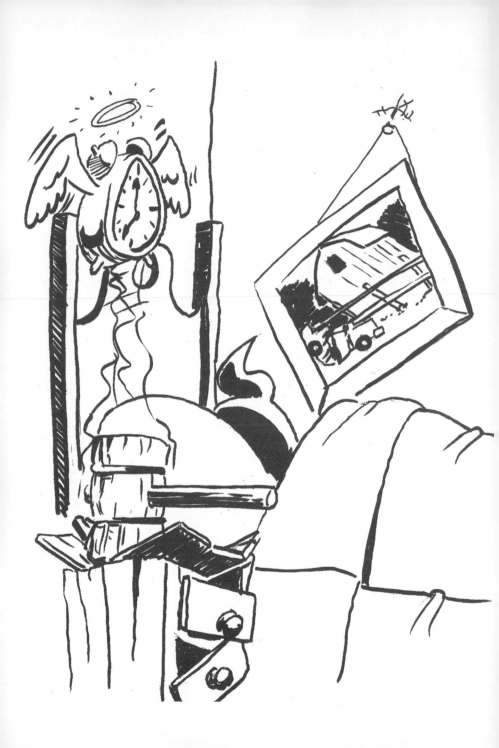

Have the front desk give you a wake-up call.

Seriously, try using more than one alarm. When you get home from work, set the alarms. Do not wait until you are sleepy. If one of your alarm clocks doesn't work, replace it. If you live with someone who normally gets up before or when you do, ask him to check on you in the morning to make sure that you are awake. Sometimes animals make pretty good alarm clocks. I have heard of cats and dogs that jump on their owner's bed at the same time everyday. Lastly, you could move into the flight path of an airport, if you are a compulsive oversleeper. I have a client who is awoken the same time everyday by the first morning flight.

If you miss your morning workout, do it later in the day or after work. You non-morning people will probably find it much more enjoyable and practical, anyhow.

 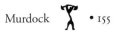

65

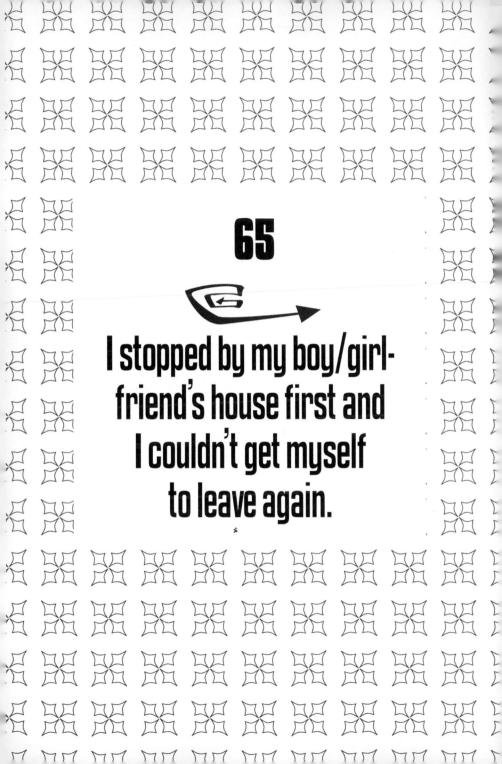

I stopped by my boy/girl-
friend's house first and
I couldn't get myself
to leave again.

←——————→

If you want to be with your honey so badly, take him along with you. Go for a walk together and you will be able to get two things done at once—exercising and talking! Consider joining a gym with your mate, so that you can motivate each other and spend more time together. It will be difficult for one person to slack off if the other person is being consistent. You will be a great influence on each other.

Complete your workout before going to his house. He should be a priority, but so should your health. If he does not understand why you need to workout first or why you need to leave his house to workout, dump him. Someone else who exercises will understand and will not make you feel guilty for taking care of yourself.

Obviously, if you do not have a boyfriend, you will not be able to use this excuse, but keep this in mind for the future. Choose a mate who exercises or would like to start now that you are around. Imagine what will happen if you take good care of yourself and your mate does not. You get married; you live a healthy lifestyle and he does not; decades later, you must take him to **chemotherapy** or cardiac rehabilitation and play nurse for the rest of his life. You wouldn't have any time for yourself, thanks to marrying someone who has unhealthy habits. Not a pretty picture is it? The sad thing is, it happens all of the time.

 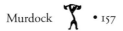

66

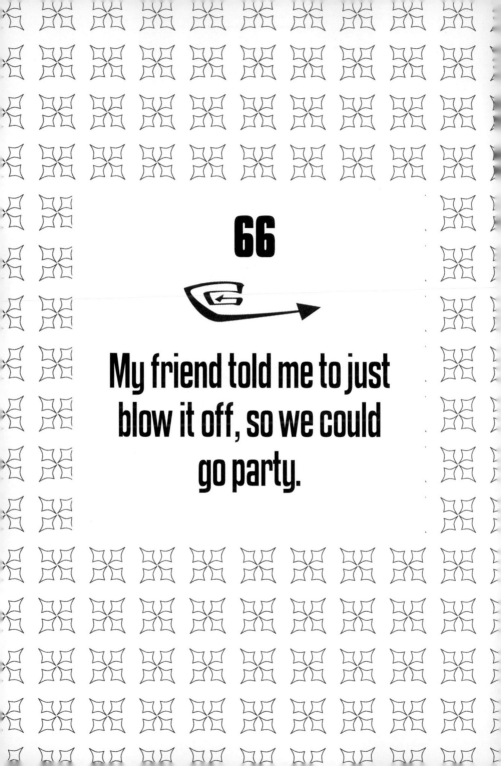

My friend told me to just blow it off, so we could go party.

This response is not too different from the previous one; please re-read it.

Choose your friends carefully. Choose friends who care about their health and yours. Good friends do not try to steer you away from what is best for you.

You do not have to choose one or the other. Ask your friend to wait for you to workout; maybe you two can go a little bit later than planned. If your friend insists on going earlier than you are able, tell her that you will just meet her at the party after your workout.

There are advantages to exercising before partying. One is that you might be less likely to drink. You might feel too well and not want to lose the high. If you do decide to drink, you will be less likely to store the Calories as fat, since your metabolism will be higher than it is at rest. Third, you might have renewed energy that is helpful when there is a long night ahead of you.

 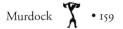

67

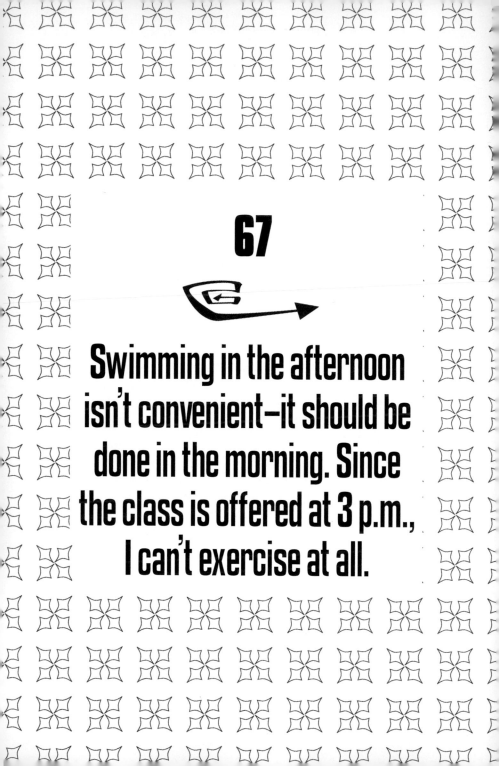

Swimming in the afternoon isn't convenient–it should be done in the morning. Since the class is offered at 3 p.m., I can't exercise at all.

Oh, please. Look around for other classes being offered. There should be plenty, since swimming is popular and an excellent form of exercise. Call the YMCA's, YWCA's, recreation centers, health clubs, high schools and colleges in your area. If you live in a complex where there is a pool, ask the manager to hire an instructor to teach the residents. Each person may need to pay for the class, or if you are lucky, the complex will pay for it.

If afternoon classes are all you can find, then make exercising in the afternoon convenient. Revise your schedule so that you can exercise. You know you would make necessary changes if you had a doctor's appointment.

There is not one particular time of day that exercise should be done. I have heard some say that exercise should be done in the afternoon, because your body temperature is higher than in the morning, according to your circadian rhythm (26). I have heard others say afternoons are better because more heart attacks occur in the morning than any other time of day (26). The best time to exercise is when you will do it. The more restrictions people have, the less likely they are to exercise.

As a last resort, choose another form of exercise. Do not give in so easily. You need the exercise.

The best time to exercise is when you will do it.

- Jeanne "Bean" Murdock

 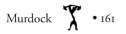

68

I'm too depressed.

Research suggests that exercise can improve psychological states, including depression. Any form of exercise like strength training and stretching can be used.

"In well-designed studies the benefits of a regular exercise program were found to be *equal to or even better than* standard forms of psychological counseling for patients with moderate depression" (20,33). "Properly supervised exercise is also a safe activity for most people using antidepressant medicine, although some medications can decrease exercise capacity" (33).

State anxiety can be reduced and positive mood factors can be elevated with even a single aerobic exercise session (38). At the same time, reductions in blood pressure and muscle tension are noticed. Brain wave patterns suggesting positive emotions occur after exercising (37).

You do not need to become an elite athlete to notice improved mood after exercising. "This is consistent with recent theories (44) that propose that changes in self-perception of fitness, rather than actual fitness improvements, are enough to enhance self-esteem or reduce depression and anxiety" (39). Therefore, fitness improvements are not required in order to enhance mental health.

 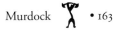

69

I forgot how to get/I got lost on my way to the gym.

Join a gym that you can see from your home or office so you will never get lost.

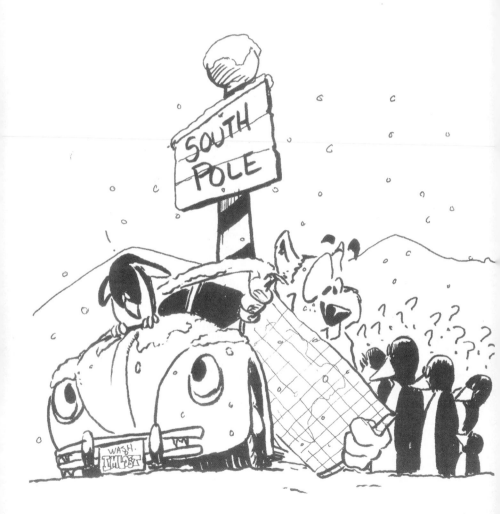

Write directions and bring them with you. Keep them in your gym bag or the glove compartment of your car. Have the gym's phone number on the same paper in case you need further assistance.

Stop at a phone booth and call the gym for directions. Do not just go home.

Join a gym that you can see from your home or office so you will never get lost.

If you spend so much time that the gym is closed by the time you get there, just go home and exercise.

Have an exercise partner who can find his way with a map and a compass. Have someone like that in the car with you and you will get anywhere you want in the most direct way possible.

 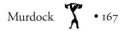

70

I was daydreaming (of how to get out of exercising) and I missed my exit.

That is OK. In the future, take the next exit and back track your way to the gym. I have done that plenty of times for various destinations, but I still go to them (after some bitching). I am sure arriving at the gym five minutes later than you had planned would not be the end of the world. It will still be there. Do not punish yourself by missing your workout—you know exercise is worth any hassle. Everyone makes mistakes.

Find ways to snap out of daydreaming, so that you do not miss your workout, again. Think about the benefits of exercise, a cute person at the gym, or the guilt you will feel if you do not go. Before you leave for the gym, set an alarm to go off just before you get to your exit. It will be sure to wake you. Ask the gym to buy billboard advertising in a place just before the exit. It would not only be a great marketing tactic, but also remind you of where you should be going.

You can always exercise at or around home. Just be sure to begin right when you arrive before you start some other project or sit for a while. Remember that variety is important. Restricting yourself to the same exercise mode will put you at a greater risk for injury than if you cross-trained.

 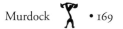

71

I got home, saw ants everywhere, and spent all my time cleaning them up.

The ants have probably been there for a while, anyway, right? What difference would it make if they are there 20, 30, or 60 minutes more? None at all. You can spray them before exercising, and then clean up when you get back. After you exercise, you will probably feel relaxed and less likely to perceive the situation as stressful. Or walk, skate, or ride to the store, if you do not have any bug spray, and get two things done at once.

When something unexpected like this arises, compromise another part of your life, not exercise. Save your laundry, cleaning (besides ants), letter writing, bill writing (gladly) for another day. Take care of yourself. Eat healthy and exercise. These habits will help you get through stressful situations and leave you with self-respect.

 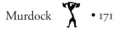

72

It was big trash
pick up day* and
I had to clean up the yard.

* when the garbage trucks will take
any amount/type of trash

This is not a bad excuse, actually. Cleaning up the yard counts as exercise, but should not replace your workouts too often. Nothing can replace strength training, which should be done two to three times a week, according to the ACSM Guidelines (4). It can help improve bone density, muscle strength and endurance, agility, coordination, and indirectly help with fat loss, by raising the metabolism. Strength training is when a resistance is so great that it cannot be moved more than fifteen times. Therefore, exercises like stair climbing, walking, or yardwork do not apply, because the intensity is light enough to do for a prolonged period of time.

Yardwork can replace cardiovascular exercise, but not often, because it is probably a lower intensity then what you usually do. You will lose some of your cardiovascular endurance, by not elevating your heart rate to the usual level. When you let yardwork replace an aerobic workout, be sure to stretch afterward, especially if yardwork is an infrequent activity for you. In addition to helping prevent muscle soreness, stretching improves range of motion, flexibility, and athletic performance. Stretching should be performed everyday, preferably after each workout.

 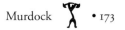

73

My make-up ran out so
I couldn't go to the gym.

Well, go chase after it.

This is another "Oh, please." If this is your excuse, you really do need to go to the gym. Remember that exercise helps to improve self-esteem. It would be a good idea to take a self-esteem workshop, too.

Think about it. You rely on make-up so much that you even have to wear it to the gym. That is not healthy. Wearing it while you are exercising is not healthy, either, because it does not allow your pores to open like they need to so that heat, water, and some electrolytes [Sodium (Na^+), Potassium (K^+), and Chloride (Cl^-)] can escape. If heat and water do not escape, you can get heat cramps, heat exhaustion, or heat stroke. If the electrolytes do not exit with the water, your blood will have too high of a concentration of them.

Maybe you wear make-up, because you have acne. Trying to cover up acne makes acne look even more noticeable. Usually there are bigger blotches of concealer where there is acne. Secondly, maybe you have skin problems *because* you wear make-up, which clogs the pores that are trying to open during exercise. It is a good idea to wash your face before and after exercise, so that your pores function properly. Consult a dermatologist, if you are an adult with acne (**rosacea**).

If you will not go to the gym or outside without make-up, exercise in your home. Dance, walk the stairs, or walk or jog in place.

74

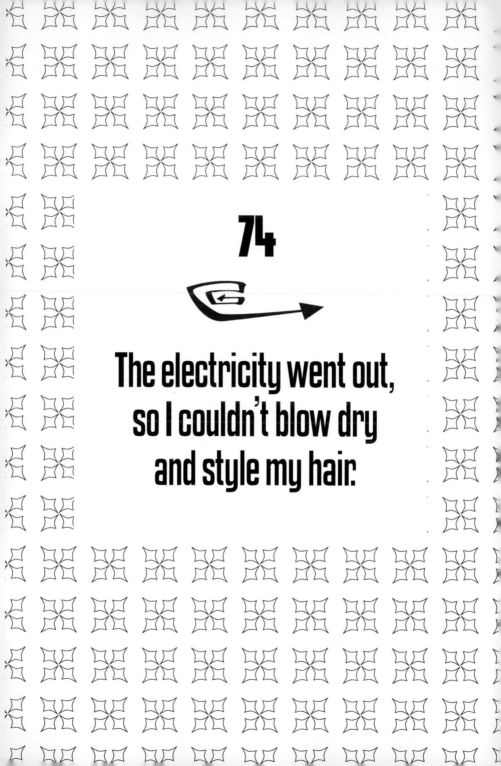

The electricity went out, so I couldn't blow dry and style my hair.

Invest in a butane hair dryer and butane curling iron. Then you will not only solve this problem, but also have two appliances that you can bring with you when traveling to foreign countries. You will not need to worry about the type of outlets they use.

Another option is to do you hair outside by your car. When the electricity goes out next time, hook up one end of jumper cables to your car battery and the other to your hair dryer or curling iron.* You will also save time by warming up your car doing your hair at the same time. Be sure your hands are dry, before trying this.

It probably would not work to use a neighbor's outlet, because her electricity would probably be out, too.

If you are intent on doing your hair first, sneak into the gym incognito and borrow a hair dryer or curling iron, or stop by a hair salon.

You really do not need to look beautiful before going to the gym, do you? Similar to the previous excuse, you might want to work on your self-esteem, too. Hopefully, you like how you look even without a hair-do. Maybe you want to meet someone while exercising, but don't you want him or her to like how you look when you are at your worst? This is a great way to weed out the bad ones. Imagine how well you would feel if you were sweaty and sloppy from exercising and someone came up to talk to you and found you attractive. What a compliment that would be.

Why not take a shower after you go to the gym, anyway? Then, you can make your impression after exercising.

*Do not try this. It is a joke!

 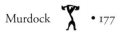

75

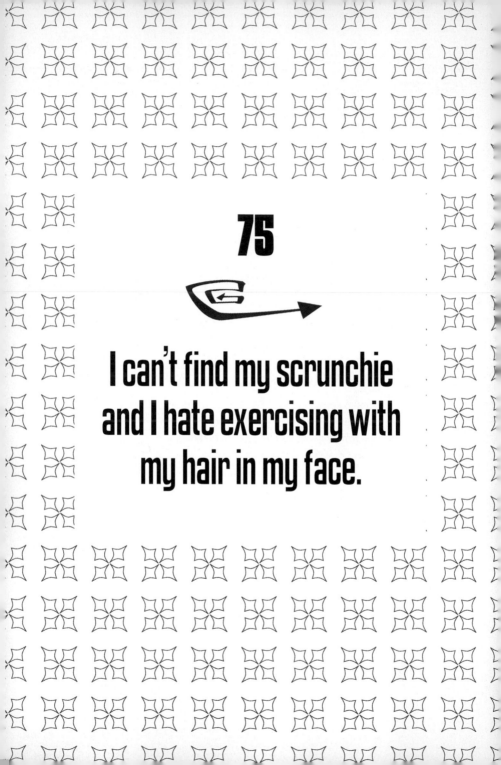

I can't find my scrunchie and I hate exercising with my hair in my face.

Baseball hats and visors work great.

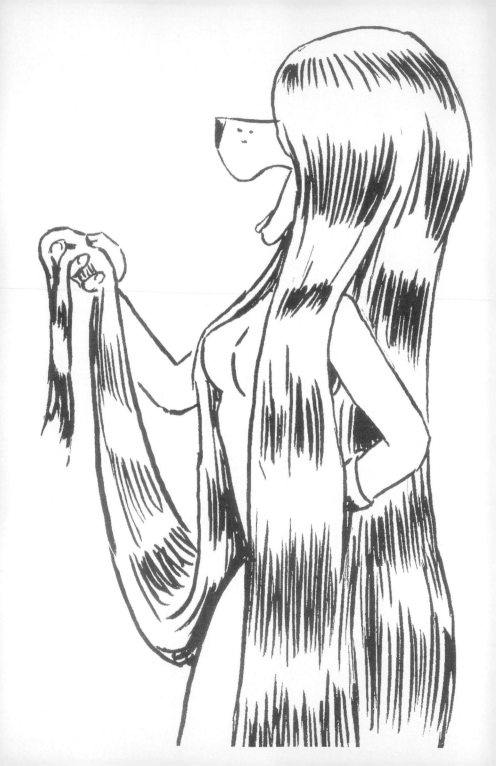

Try using a rubber band. It is not stylish and it will pull out half your hair when you take it off, but at least your hair will not be in your face.

Baseball hats and visors work great. If you have a hat, make sure it has a mesh or thin lining, otherwise you will get too hot. You do not want to retain too much of the (approximately) 50% body heat that is normally lost through your head. Hats not only keep your hair out of your face, but also they seem to be fashionable now. The disadvantage of using a scrunchie is that it can hurt your head when you are exercising on your back. It can get in the way when doing exercises like the lat pull down, where a weight machine's horizontal bar is brought behind your head to the base of the neck. A hat solves those two problems.

If your hair is long enough to be put in a scrunchie, it should be long enough to tie in a knot. Roll your hair up as though it were to be put in a bun. Then, take the end of your hair and put it in through the center of the circle you just made. It works.

As a last resort, you can cut your hair.

 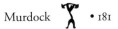

76

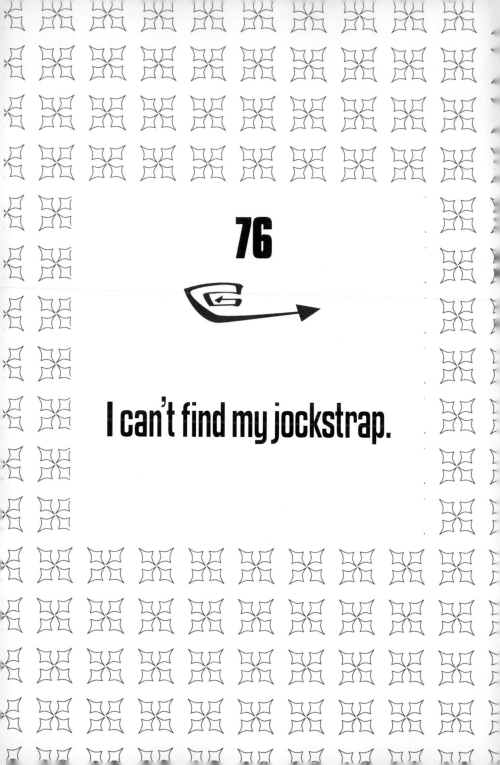

I can't find my jockstrap.

⟵—————⟶

Did you look . . . ? OK. This is a tough one for me. I do not know where one would put a jockstrap after being used. Fortunately, I have never needed to wear one. Just look everywhere. At least you did not say, "My dog ate my jockstrap."

Forget about the strap for now and just do a low intensity workout that will not create a lot of jarring. Exercising at a low intensity long duration would add variety to your routine, anyway. If you are more worried about how you look, keep the spandex tights at home or wear shorts or sweats over them.

 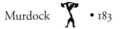

77

I just got my hair done.

Bad timing. If you were exercising daily, any day would be bad timing, actually.

Try exercising differently from how you normally do. Stay indoors if you normally go outdoors. Exercise in a gym or at home, so the weather will not mess up your hair. Exercise at a lower intensity than you normally do, even if it is a leisurely walk on the treadmill. It is really important that you still do something, so that you can stay in the habit and routine that you have created.

For swimmers, do deep-water running and exercises with an AquaJogger™ or shallow-water running and exercises. They both keep your head dry and out of the water. If you have long hair, clip it up.

Tell your hair stylist to have recumbent (like sitting in a chair) bicycles in her shop, instead of barber chairs. Ride the bike while waiting your turn or while sitting underneath a dryer. By the time your hair is done, your workout will be, too.

 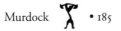

78

I just got my nails done.

Not a problem. Deciding how to get around this excuse depends on whether you are concerned about the nails not being dry, yet, or having them broken. If you are concerned about the former, choose an exercise that does not require you to hold anything like walking, stationary biking, stair climbing (if you can do it without holding on), aerobics, or dancing. Being outside or in a gym exercising would even help your nails dry quickly, due to fresh air or typical dry, cool air in a gym. You may incorporate waving your hands into an exercise routine. In different directions, move your arms at your elbow and shoulder joints—calisthenics for the arms! If you have very high blood pressure (high b.p. > 145/95 mm Hg), be careful about raising your arms above your head, because your exercising blood pressure may go higher (too high is > 260/115 mm Hg) than is healthy. Note: it is normal for the first number (systolic) to elevate during exercise, and for the second number (diastolic) to stay about the same or decrease.

If you are concerned about your nails breaking, well, you will just need to take a chance. You will always need to exercise despite any excuse or fear, so do not hold back. If you break a nail while exercising, you will pay less to get it fixed than you would for open-heart surgery. Sedentary lifestyle is one of the four primary risk factors for heart disease; the other three being smoking, high blood pressure, and high cholesterol.

Wear baseball batting gloves when strength training. They have long enough fingers to protect the nails and will help prevent calluses.

 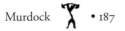

79

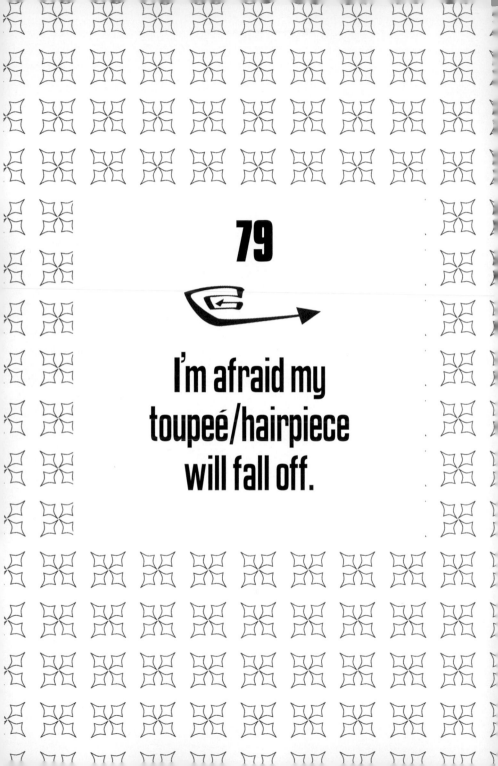

I'm afraid my toupeé/hairpiece will fall off.

If you live in Chicago, it probably would not be a good idea to exercise outdoors. Although, you could wear a baseball hat, which will also keep the sun out of your eyes in the summer and keep your head warm in the winter. In the summer, make sure the hat has a mesh lining so that heat can escape from your head, thereby keeping your body temperature normal.

Try not wearing your hairpiece at all. Then you do not have to worry about it falling off. Surely you have heard that bald is beautiful?

Have you considered hair transplantation?*

Choose an exercise that does not involve a lot of jarring. Exercise at a lower intensity and a longer duration than you would otherwise. For example, instead of jogging at 5 m.p.h. for 20 minutes, walk at 4 m.p.h. for 30 minutes. Strength training is not a jarring exercise (if it is for you, you are doing it wrong), but there could be times when you need to be leaning over or lying down. A baseball hat would be helpful in this situation, too. It will keep your hair in place and prevent others from seeing that the hair is not real (a concern for some people). You could even wear a hat instead of a hairpiece.

As for swimming, you could wear a bathing cap to conceal your bald head.

*I neither recommend nor discourage it.

 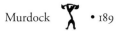

80

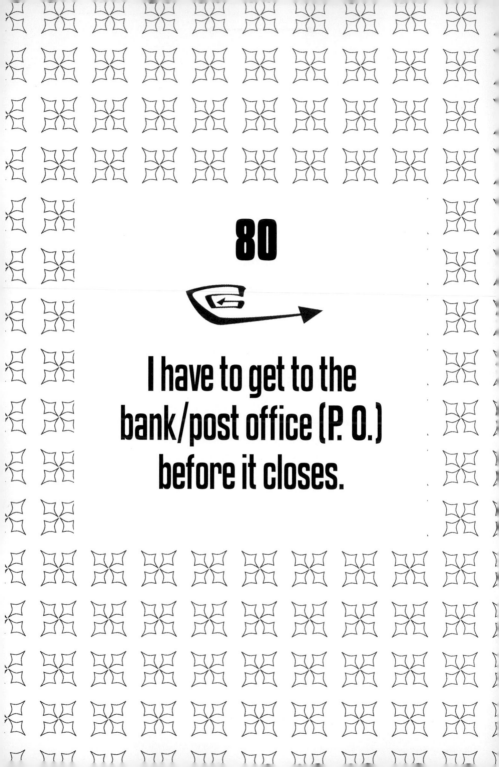

I have to get to the
bank/post office (P. O.)
before it closes.

This is another occasion when time management skills are helpful. Plan your time better, so that you are not only not rushing to the bank or P. O., but also getting to exercise. You can accomplish both at the same time—walk, bike, or skate to the bank or P. O. Choose a bank or P. O. close to your home or office so that you can get there without a car.

Why have I never heard someone say, "I can't do _____, because I have to get to the gym before it closes"? Make exercise a top priority! Make your health a top priority!

If you drive to the bank or P. O., exercise afterward. Rushing to the bank should mean that it would not be taking much time to do the errand. You will have plenty of time to exercise, still.

Take advantage of the bank's convenient services like direct deposit and automated tellers. Sign up with your employer to have your paycheck directly deposited into your bank account, which usually happens the night before your payday. When you need some cash, use the automated teller and don't worry about the bank's hours.

Go to the bank or P. O. during one of your breaks, so that it's not so near to closing time. Then you can exercise after work. Most banks and P. O.'s are open on Saturdays, so you can go then instead of during the week.

 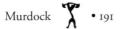

81

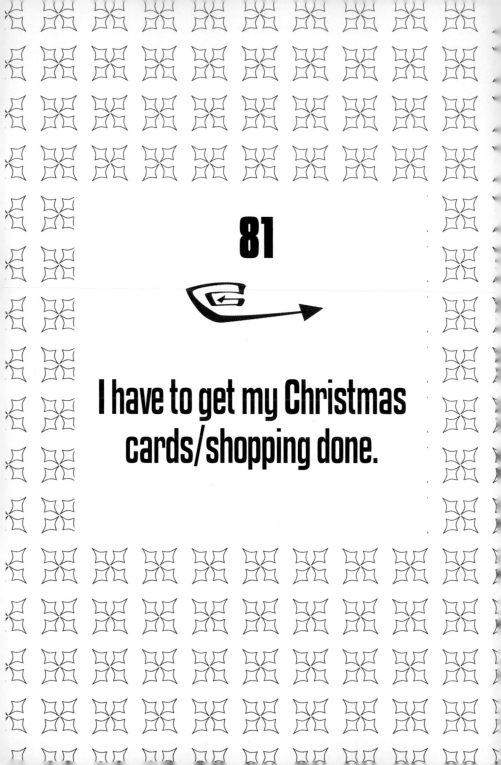

I have to get my Christmas cards/shopping done.

It is great that you are keeping in touch with your friends and relatives and wanting to write them, but it cannot supersede exercise. You are being a good role model by sending Christmas cards. Become a role model by exercising too. Exercising can not only improve your self-esteem, but also improve how others perceive you. I have a lot of respect for people who take care of themselves.

Start on your cards and shopping after Thanksgiving, doing a little at a time, so that each day you have time to exercise, too. Waiting until the last minute will not only make the holidays a chore, but also stressful.

Use your shopping time as a way to exercise. Park your car in the back of the lot and climb stairs and escalators instead of using elevators. Choose larger malls with multiple levels in which to shop, so that you can walk more. Carry out your own groceries from a supermarket rather than having a bag boy help you. Go to a shopping center that has a gym where you can workout before or after shopping. You will save time by not driving to several areas. Take your purchases out to your car instead of having a store hold onto them for you. Hide the purchases in the trunk out of sight from thieves.

Before starting your Christmas cards, exercise. Once you get on a roll with writing, you may not want to stop. You can also use exercise as a nice break from writing, which will make you feel relaxed and clear-minded.

 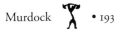

82

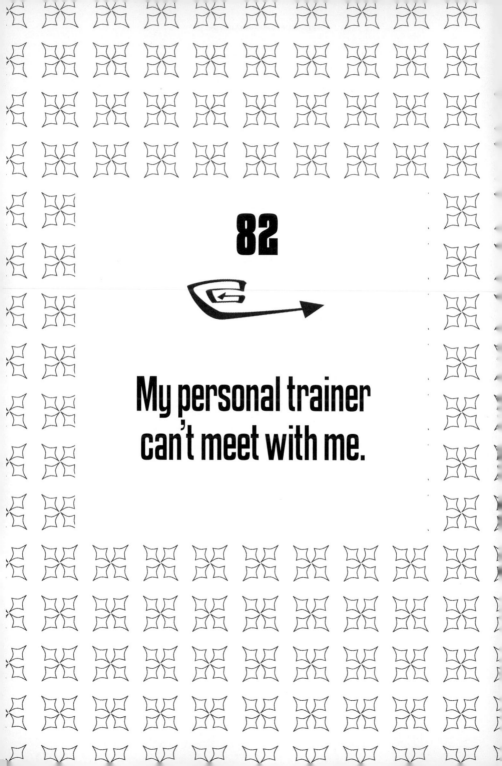

My personal trainer can't meet with me.

Of course I think it is great that you have a coach, but he should be helping you to be independent, too. You should know the name, form, and number of sets and repetitions of each strength training exercise. It is nice to have someone tell you what to do, but you need to be prepared for exercising on your own, like in this instance. I give an explanation for everything that I suggest, so that my clients not only understand their routines, but also can logically figure out what to do when I am not with them. For example, I teach how to know what weight to use and when to change repetitions.

A trainer is a motivator, too. This is when a friend comes in handy. When your trainer cannot meet with you, ask a friend to workout with you. Even if she does not know a lot about strength training, she can encourage you. It also makes the workout more interesting. It would be a good chance to see her and catch up on the latest gossip. That's real quality time, getting to workout with a friend rather than going out drinking together.

It is very important that your trainer does not tell you to skip your workout. You need to do whatever it takes to stay on your schedule; even if that means choosing a different exercise mode or workout than you usually do. Missing a workout can have a domino effect—just skip one day, just skip two days, just skip three days; you know how hard it is to start again. Also, it is important that you do not wait more than five days between strength training sessions or you will start losing what you had worked so hard to gain. If you do not use the muscles often enough they forget what to do, and your trainer will need to have you work easier than the previous session, so that you do not hurt yourself.

 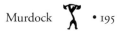

83

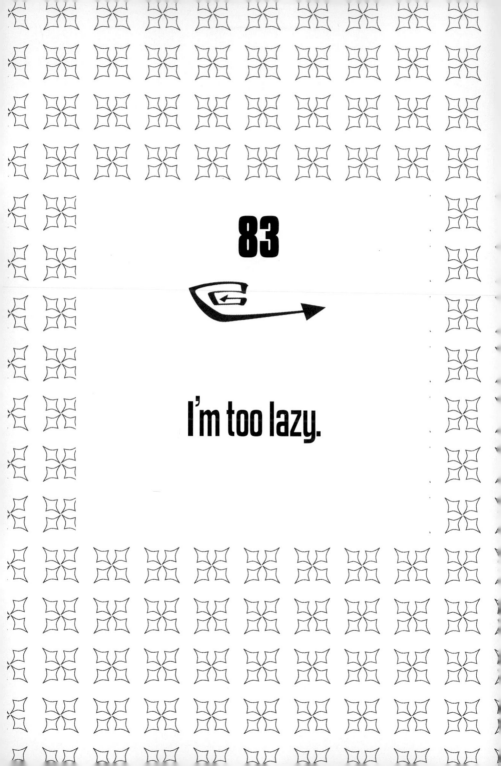

I'm too lazy.

Well, I am not surprised. We do live in an automatic everything society. We push a button to open the garage, to turn on the TV or DVD player, to cook our food, and to wash our laundry. If there were a pill invented that could replace exercise, it would make a billion dollars. The 75% of Americans who do not engage in regular physical activity would probably buy it.

According to the Journal of the American Medical Association (30), "in the period 1988 to 1991, 33.4% of U. S. adults 20 years of age or older were estimated to be overweight. Comparisons of the 1988 to 1991 overweight prevalence estimates with data from earlier surveys indicate dramatic increases in all race/sex groups. Overweight prevalence increased 8% between the 1976 to 1980 and 1988 to 1991 surveys. During this period, for adult men and women aged 20 through 74 years, . . . mean body weight increased 3.6 kg" (7.92 lbs.). During the period 1999-2002, it was estimated that 65% of U. S. adults were overweight and 30% (about half of the 65%) were obese. As for children and adolescents (6-19 years old), 16% were overweight (22). Avoid becoming part of these statistics. If you are already overweight, do something about it. Start exercising today. Even for just ten minutes.

Laziness can be good, though. It is good for avoiding the 101 benefits of exercise, listed in the beginning of this book. Laziness can get you a heart attack, cancer, osteoporosis, and low self-esteem. There's no effort, and it is free!

Seriously, do not find yourself on a hospital bed with tubes coming out of you after open-heart surgery, wishing you had made an effort earlier in life to take care of yourself. It takes much more effort to lower you cholesterol, increase bone density, improve your mood, and control diabetes through exercise than it does to prevent them. It is easier to use exercise to *prevent* a problem than it is to *treat* a problem. Do not let laziness poison you, jeopardize your standard of living, or bring you to an early grave.

It is easier to use exercise to *prevent* a problem than it is to *treat* a problem.
- Jeanne "Bean" Murdock

 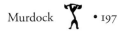

84

It's that time of the month/I'm PMS-ing.

Exercise can help relieve and even prevent the symptoms of pre-menstrual syndrome (PMS).

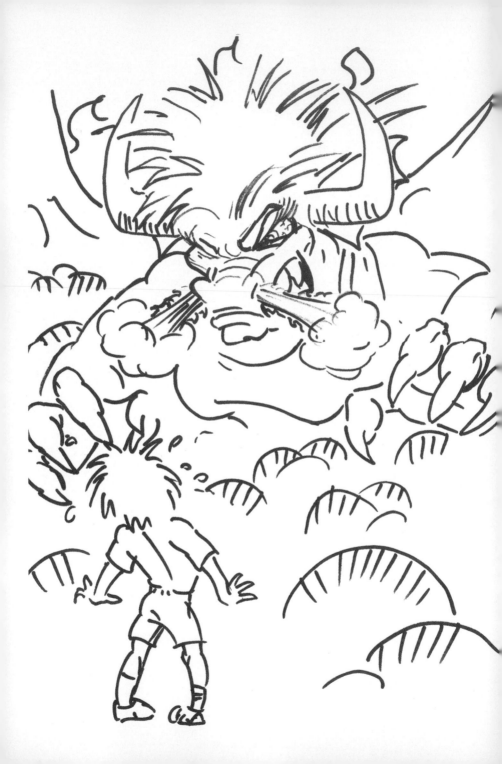

Exercise can help relieve and even prevent the symptoms of pre-menstrual syndrome (PMS). It can help combat mild depression and may stimulate the release of **endorphins**, pain relieving molecules. "A 1993 Duke University study compared a group of women who did aerobic exercise for one hour three times a week with a group who did strength training. PMS symptoms improved to some degree for all the women, but the aerobic group reaped especially significant benefits, particularly for depression" (47).

If you were part of the 20% of women who exercise vigorously, you would not have to worry about it being that time of the month. You, in addition to half of all elite female athletes, would be amenorrheic (without menstrual cycles) (25). This is not healthy, though, because it can lead to endometrial cancer, osteoporosis, scoliosis (curvature of the spine), and infertility. It is thought that amenorrhea results from altered hormone production associated with a high volume of exercise and low Caloric intake.

This is the opposite extreme of not exercising at all, but it shows that you should find a happy medium. By exercising moderately, you may find that you have decreased blood flow during menstruation, less cramping, little if any PMS, longer cycles, fewer days of menstruation, and less low back pain, headaches, anxiety, depression, and fatigue. More research needs to be done on the effects of exercise on PMS and menstrual symptoms, because the current studies have shown contradicting results.

Since some women have even reported a worsening of symptoms during exercise, workout at a low intensity and short duration at first. Test how your body reacts to exercise during menstruation, increasing the effort gradually if your body approves. It is worth a try.

85

I have too much
cooking to do.

Turn on your favorite music and exercise while you cook. Walk or jog in place or dance around the kitchen. You may have some free time while something is in the oven or on the stove, but you cannot leave the house. That is understandable. Climb the stairs in your home for a few minutes, hop on your stationary bike or treadmill, or continue dancing.

If you have a bicycle and enjoy riding it, but find a lot of occasions when you cannot leave the house, get a stationary trainer. Companies like Trek®, Minoura, and Giant® make these, which enable you to take the front tire off of your bike and connect it to a stationary stand. The back wheel of the bike is also on part of the stand. It is a better investment than a stationary bike, if you already have a street bicycle. You should be able to find the stands at any bike shop.

Try exercising before you start cooking, even if it is just for 15 minutes. It would be to your advantage, because you will probably find that exercise will suppress your appetite. You will be less likely to snack on what you are cooking.

You may have someone around who can watch the food cooking for 10 minutes at a time. That is very useful. Go out for two or three 10-minute bouts of exercise. If the bouts are at the same intensity as one 20- or 30-minute session, you will benefit the same. "DeBusk and colleagues compared the effects of one 30-minute bout versus three 10-minute bouts of walking/jogging per day performed at 65 to 75 percent of maximum heart rate, five times per week for eight weeks, in 40 previously sedentary middle aged men" (11). They found that both groups significantly increased their cardiovascular endurance and were able to lose weight similarly (about 1.76 kg or 3.87 lbs.).

 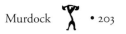

86

It's hunting/fishing season.

Choose the type of river, creek or ocean fishing where you can stand in the water. Having to walk in deep water and cast your line is great exercise. Make a point to walk along the shore for a few minutes at a time, then cast the line. It would not only give you a good opportunity to find the perfect spot, but also make you less tired from simply standing. This is true for casting from land, too. Walking aids in blood circulation thereby preventing pooling in your legs. Varicose (bulging) veins can even occur in people who are on their feet (standing) for several hours at a time. The veins bulge because their damaged valves cause the blood to flow too slowly or to backflow.

Deep sea fishermen: Take frequent breaks from sitting. Walk or jog around the boat or in place for 10 minutes at a time. It will break up the monotony when the bites are few and far between and you will get your exercise for the day.

Lake fishermen who are in a boat or canoe should paddle out to the middle of the lake. It is great exercise and you will not scare the fish away from you. Once you are out there, take a few breaks by paddling some more.

Hunting can be great exercise, too, so use it to your advantage. I have heard of people putting in a few miles worth of hiking to reach the animals' location. Even before the season starts, you may spend several weeks staking out the prey. Do your homework so that you can exercise and get your perfect shot, too. (By the way, I am not necessarily supporting hunting).

 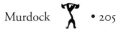

87

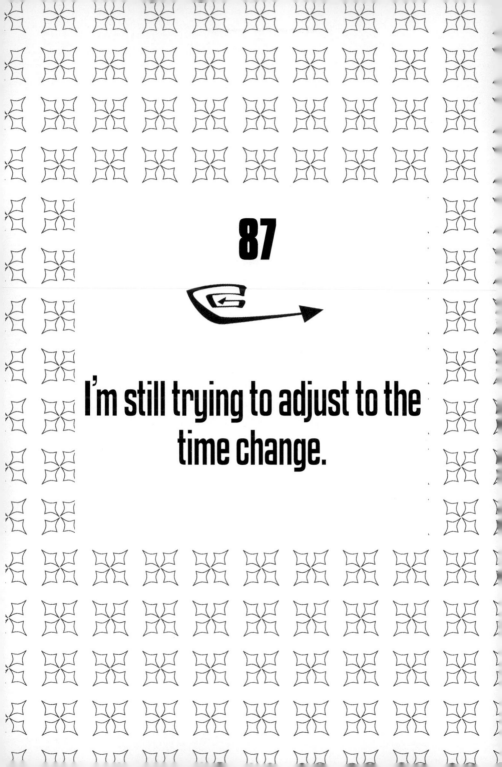

I'm still trying to adjust to the time change.

Exercise now. Exercise can help you to adjust to the change. If you had been exercising consistently before the time changed, you may not have even felt the physiological effects at all. I know I never have. (This does not mean that you necessarily will not.) The time change may affect your circadian rhythm, but it is no reason to avoid exercise. You may feel more tired at times of the day when you are normally not, or even all day long. Exercise could give you more energy, so workout before your new lull in the day and you may avoid it. Plan to exercise two or three times, 10-15 minutes each, throughout the day to keep your metabolism higher than normal and keep you energetic. If you won't have time for two or three sessions in a day, exercise once for a longer period of time.

Next time that we are supposed to adjust our clocks, make a point to exercise at least a couple of weeks in advance. Better yet, start exercising, now, and stay consistent. You'll find that you can handle all types of changes better than you used to. These include changes that affect you psychologically, too, such as moving, changing jobs, death in the family, divorce, and even positive changes like promotions. Positive and negative changes create stress. As I discuss in excuse number 120, exercise can help to alleviate, if not prevent, a situation from being perceived as stressful.

 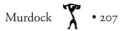

88

I'm waiting until daylight savings time.

So, you only exercise six months out of the year? What if you lived in the very northern part of the world where they have few hours of sunlight? When would you make time for exercise? Are you waiting until daylight savings time, because you need it to stay lighter out longer or do you just feel better during this time? As discussed in excuse number 32, you can still exercise when it is dark, whether in the early morning or at night. Just take the necessary precautions, like wearing reflective clothing, to be safe. Exercise year-round and you will feel well year-round, not just six months out of the year.

When daylight savings time arrives and you start exercising, will you continue for the whole six months? If not, you will need to write down what other excuses you are using, then review my responses to those.

Even if you do exercise consistently for the whole six months, you will reap the benefits only during that time. They will not carry over until the next daylight savings time. Every time you stop exercising, you lose everything you had gained, and then you have to start from scratch again. If you want to live a long, healthy lifestyle, you need to exercise consistently.

 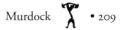

89

My horoscope says that this is not a good time in my life to be exercising.

Your horoscope is correct, if you want to live an unhealthy lifestyle. If that is the case, your horoscope may as well say that this is a good time in your life to have a heart attack, or be diagnosed with cancer, tear a muscle carrying groceries, sprain (overstretch or tear of a ligament) your ankle stepping off a curb.

Exercise can not only help to prevent diseases, but also injuries. Being on an exercise program that includes cardiovascular exercise, strength training, and stretching, will strengthen your heart and other muscles, and increase muscle flexibility. The stronger and more agile your muscles are, the less chance there is that you will tear one.

I helped rehabilitate a client's knee after he injured it running up a flight of stairs. If he had been on an exercise program before the stair run, the injury probably would not have occurred. When the muscles are untrained, they become weaker, smaller, tighter, and more prone to injuries. The same is true for tendons, which connect muscle to bone, and ligaments, which connect bone to bone.

For those of you who religiously read your horoscopes, collect a few days or weeks worth. Line them up and see how many of the predictions were accurate. This should guide your decision in whether or not to take them seriously or just to have fun with them, a lighthearted approach. Remember that horoscopes are not based on scientific evidence—exercise is!

90

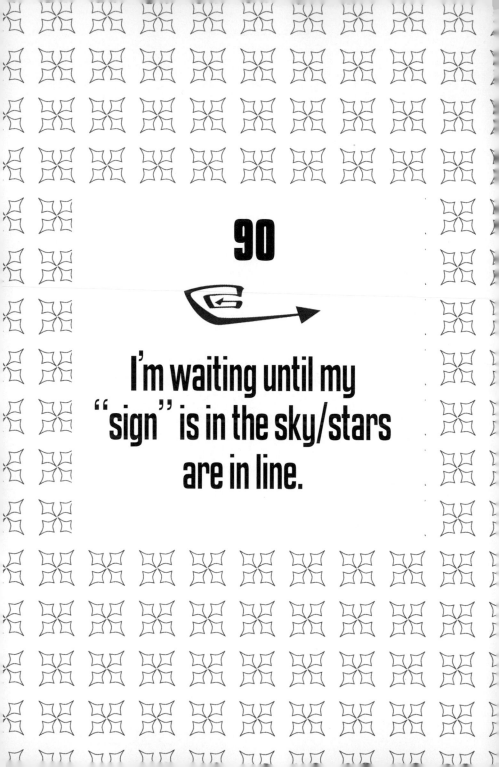

I'm waiting until my "sign" is in the sky/stars are in line.

If the sign for which you are waiting says, "Get your butt in gear and start exercising," I hope that it comes along, soon. The longer you wait to start exercising, the more your body will deteriorate, the harder it will be to start, and the longer it will take to get in shape. From what I know about astrology, signs are in the sky only sometimes. That would mean you only exercise sometimes. Part of taking care of yourself includes exercising about five days a week for at least 30 minutes. This needs to be done consistently for the rest of your life, not just sometimes.

Waiting until the stars are in line is not a bad idea if they are at a gym's front door, before opening time. Are we talking about a Hollywood gym where all of the big names go? Maybe we are talking about Gym Milky Way? Seriously, do not wait to start exercising. Just like I wrote for excuse number 89, we need to workout now for the rest of our lives. Start an exercise program and continue until death. Otherwise, sit and watch the people around you living an independent lifestyle.

 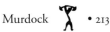

91

God had to rest, too, you know.

From what I know about religion, which is very little, God worked hard for six days before resting. It was not just work work, it was manual labor. He had a lot of exercise. If you exercise very hard for six days in a row, you should rest one day, too. ONE day. You would deserve it.

It is a good idea to rest one day a week to decrease the chance of injury and burn out. I have seen a lot of people who exercise seven days a week at the onset of an exercise program and become burned out after two weeks. It is too much at first. They are wearing themselves out; they need to work up slowly to doing more exercise. Those are usually the same types of people who look at the scale at the end of the two weeks and do not see any change. Then they quit their routine. Doing too much exercise before the body is ready can lead to a misuse injury. Getting shin splints at the start of a running program is a type of misuse injury. If you are not used to walking for an extended period of time (more than 30 minutes), you should not start running. You need to work up to it slowly. A shin splint is an idiopathic (of unknown origin) pain between the ankle and the knee. It could be torn tissue around a muscle or the muscle itself that is damaged from the impact of running.

If you are the type who thinks one day off from exercising will turn into two days off, then three, etc., on the seventh day exercise at a lower intensity or less duration than you usually do. For instance, if you normally walk hills for 45 minutes, walk on a flat surface for just 20 minutes. I understand that some of you want to make exercise a daily habit and are either afraid of stopping or you like it a lot. That is OK.

Do not make your life one big rest period. Rest when you need it such as after exercising for five or six days. You do not need to exercise five or six days a week right when you start a program, but it is a good goal to have. Just do two or three days a week, for now, or just one day if that is what is practical. Have a clear goal in your mind, and on paper, and work up to it. Plan to do some physical activity almost every day of the week, eventually, for a total of 30 minutes each day. Then you, too, can rest the seventh day.

92

I have jury duty.

Courts are not in session on the weekends, so there are two days you can exercise. Secondly, court usually goes about the same hours as a typical workday, 9 a.m.-5 p.m., give or take an hour. There are usually breaks, too. Take your pick. Exercise on the weekends, lunchtime, before or after court, or during a short recess.

Whether jury duty lasts for one day or several months, you will need to put your life on hold, temporarily, but not your health. Your health always comes first. If you were conscious and thought you were having a heart attack, you would immediately admit yourself to an emergency room. You would not say that you couldn't seek help, because you have jury duty, would you? No. Of course not. Your health matters to you. Make it matter enough so that you exercise, too. Make prevention as much a priority as medical treatment. Let us prevent misfortune, like a heart attack at a young age. Exercise and proper eating habits are the ways to prevent lifestyle-related diseases and injuries.

Take advantage of the breaks you get while on jury duty. Even a ten minute walk during a break would be great! Do three of those and you have your minimum requirement for the day.

Regarding strength training, it is really important you continue to do it. You may be used to doing it as often as three times a week for an hour, but have stopped completely during jury duty. Continue. Complete your workout before or after court. Even if you do the workouts just two times a week and one set of each exercise, you still can maintain your fitness level, and even improve.

93

I won the lottery.

The healthier you are, the longer you will live, and the more time you will have to spend your winnings or earnings!

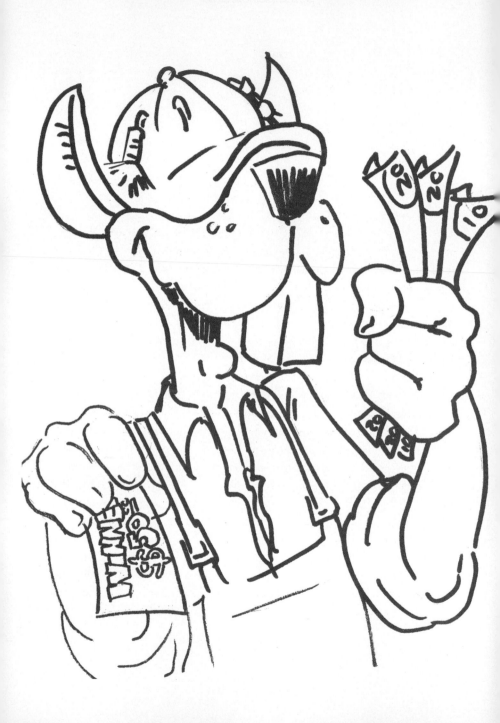

Even more reason to exercise. Now it is easier for you to afford a personal fitness trainer, all the exercise equipment you want, and even a house in which to put it. You can even afford to buy your own gym that specializes in your favorite sport or exercise. If you like baseball, you can have a batting cage on site. For those of you who like weight lifting, you can buy free weights and every piece of equipment that Cybex™ makes for physical therapy, which is more advanced than what they offer for gyms and homes.

I assume that you will not be working if you won the lottery, so you will have even more time to exercise. Just play, play, play. After you buy your ski boat, you can take up water skiing. Travel around the U. S. with your boat, being pulled by your new motor home, and ski in all of the well-known lakes. If golf is your sport, spend your time traveling around the world and playing at the fanciest courses. Be sure to walk part if not all of the course, pulling or carrying your own bag. Remember that we are finding ways to exercise regularly. Driving from hole to hole in a golf cart does not do much for the heart. If you prefer walking for exercise, spend your time sightseeing around the world. There are many walking and hiking tours available and of course sights to see and trails to walk on your own. Use travel books by Fodor® and Frommers® to plan your trips.

Have you ever wanted to be pampered at a health spa? Use your newfound money to travel around the world and to visit spas. Treat yourself to massages, facials, delicious meals, and of course plenty of exercise. The *Ultimate Spa Book* (40) outlines the top 70 spas in the world, giving arrival information, an overall rating, negative and positive aspects, the main thrust, and cost for each one. There is at least one photograph for each spa, so that you can get a better idea of the atmosphere.

One thing winning the lottery will not do for you is bestow good health. That takes a lot of hard work to achieve and maintain. No matter how rich you are, you still need to exercise, eat well, stay away from drugs including cigarettes, and control mental stress levels. What good does a million dollars do if you are too sick to use it? I guess it is good for paying hospital bills. This is the same for those of you who earned the money you have. Do not let money blind you from seeing reality. The healthier you are, the longer you will live, and the more time you will have to spend your winnings or earnings!

 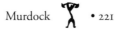

94

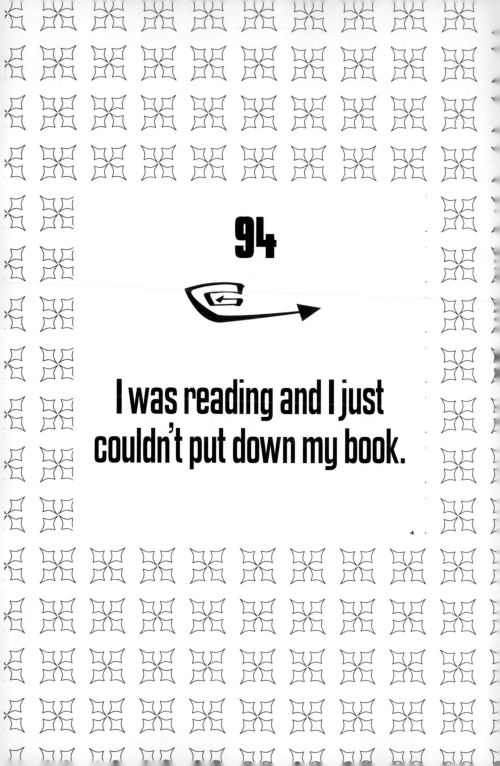

I was reading and I just couldn't put down my book.

Was it too heavy? Was it glued to your hands?

If it is this book, it's OK. Just kidding. It's NOT OK. Finish reading this excuse response and one other that best fits you, then go out and exercise. This book is not going anywhere. It will be here when you get back, unless you have a dog that likes to chew on things or a child who likes to rearrange the house. In either case, put the book out of reach.

Whether this or any other book is the one that you cannot put down, there are ways to compromise. Plan on exercising on a stairclimber, treadmill, or stationary bicycle where you can read and workout at the same time. Most of these machines either come with reading racks or have a place on which one can be put. If not, just hold your book. If you are like me, you cannot exercise and read at the same time, and you will need to put down the book and come back to it later.

I assume that you do not have time to finish the book and then exercise. So as a last resort, walk in place while you are reading. Maybe you will find the walking helps you retain more of what you read than if you were sedentary.

 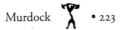

95

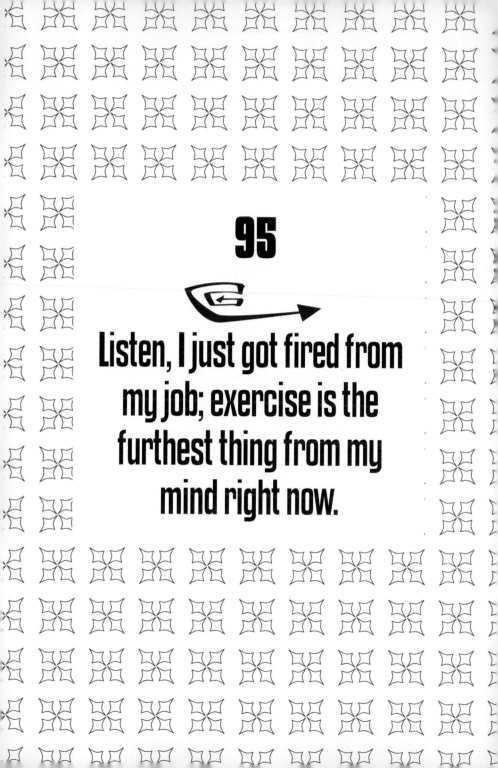

Listen, I just got fired from my job; exercise is the furthest thing from my mind right now.

This is a time when you could really use exercise. Ending a job, whether it is on a good or bad note, is one of the most stressful things that can happen to you. It may even decrease your self-esteem. As was discussed earlier in this book, exercise can help control stress and improve self-esteem, something you need when looking for a new job. Can you imagine an employer hiring someone who does not have confidence that he can do the job?

If you are out of work, you will have more time to exercise. Take advantage, by doing some things for yourself—taking care of yourself. Take some time off and do things that you had wanted to do, like hiking up the nearby mountain or hill, renting Rollerblades™, golfing, biking around town, walking with friends, or using your home exercise equipment.

Combine exercise with job hunting. Walk to the copy shop to design, copy, and fax your résumé and cover letter. Or, walk to the post office to mail your applications. Walk around business parks, to pick up and drop off applications, network, and learn more about how the companies operate. Walk, run, skate, or bike to a library where you can research companies. Carry your necessities in a backpack, when you exercise to an interview. I am sure that a potential employer would love to see that you take care of yourself. It means they will pay less for medical insurance. Drive as little as possible. Remember that you have more time to exercise and you need it.

 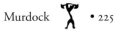

96

I got lost in my music.

Try looking between the quarter and half notes.

Bring your music with you when exercising. Carry a Sony Walkman™ or Discman™. These are great accessories to have when you need to leave the house for a workout. Get a portable radio, if your favorite music is broadcasted. Tune Belt™ makes special carrying cases for portable radios, and tape and CD players that can be worn comfortably around the waist. They are made from neoprene (wet suit material), fitting snuggly, and do not bounce around like fanny packs do.

I assume that if you exercise at home you will not use this excuse. You can play your music and exercise. If you do not normally exercise at home and are determined not to leave the house, dance to the music that you are playing. Dancing is a safe, effective, fun form of exercise that you can do at home. Taking dancing lessons to learn how to move to your favorite music can increase your exercise level.

97

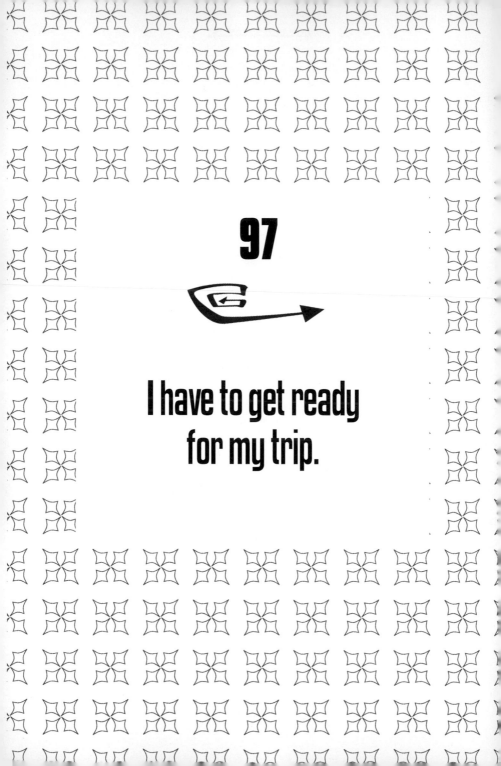

I have to get ready
for my trip.

It is a good idea to be as healthy as possible when traveling. Fit exercise into your busy schedule, by doing it before or after preparations. Take frequent exercise breaks to accumulate at least 30 minutes of exercise each day. Leave the car at home, when going to the post office to suspend mail delivery; the barber shop; the travel store to get books or maps; the travel agent to get your tickets; and a friend's house to leave your house key.

I think that the most efficient use of your time would be to make a list, while exercising, of errands to do and things to pack. Hop on a treadmill or exercise bike, or walk outside with pen and paper in hand, or walk in place at home. By the time you are done exercising, your list will be complete. You will be able to go right to your closet and quickly pack your suitcases without having to walk around in a daze wondering what to bring. You will know in what order to do your errands, on which days, and when you will have time to exercise, too. This will be the fastest you will have ever been prepared to travel.

You can also turn packing into an aerobic workout. Put on some music and dance while gathering your clothes. Run, march, or walk briskly back and forth from your dresser and closet to your suitcase. Wear what you normally would for exercising, so that you can get in the mood. Include your exercise shoes, so you decrease the impact on your joints.

Remember to pack your exercise clothes. You need to take care of yourself away from home, too.

 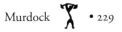

98

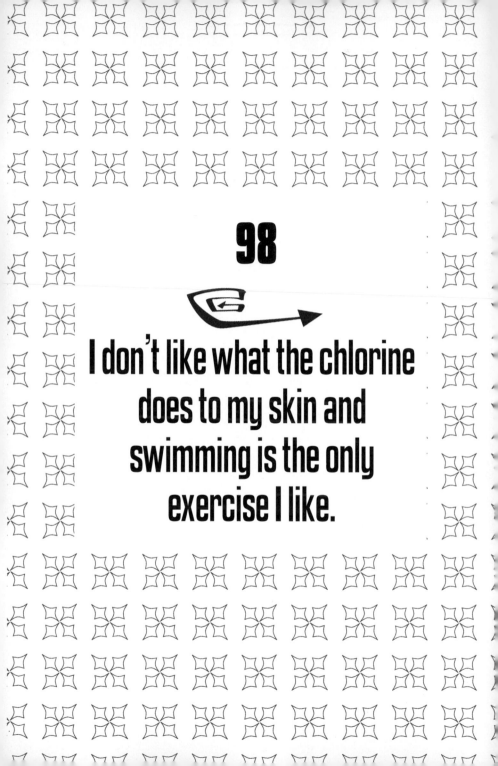

I don't like what the chlorine does to my skin and swimming is the only exercise I like.

I understand that some people are allergic to chlorine and are told by their doctors that they cannot swim in pools. I think that doctors should be very careful to whom they tell not to swim, because there are those patients who only like swimming or can only exercise in the water, for example senior citizens who have arthritis. After the doctor's warning, the patient might not exercise at all. I have seen this happen.

Work with a dermatologist and use his suggestions so that you can continue to swim. If necessary, get a second or third opinion. Do not give up on swimming. You are ahead of a lot of people who do not have any exercise at all that they enjoy.

If there is a nearby lake or ocean and you are a strong enough swimmer, consider exercising in it. Take a swimming instructor out with you the first few times, if you are nervous or are not a very strong swimmer. Afterwards, take a buddy with you in case of an emergency. Tell the lifeguard, if there is one, to keep an eye on you.

Consider getting your own pool. They are expensive, but a worthwhile investment if it's the only place you will exercise. In your own pool, you can maintain the chlorine at a tolerable level.

Try asking if the chlorine levels can be lowered where you swim. If you use a large, city pool, they will probably say no. It takes a lot of chemicals to counteract all of the bacteria brought in to a busy pool. Find a private pool or live in an apartment or condominium complex that has one. They will be more likely to accommodate you. Be realistic, though. Pool maintenance people will be using standards set for them by the health department.

As a last resort, find a new mode of exercise. You know you need to take care of yourself and that you are concerned about your skin, so try something different. It will be worth it.

 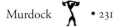

99

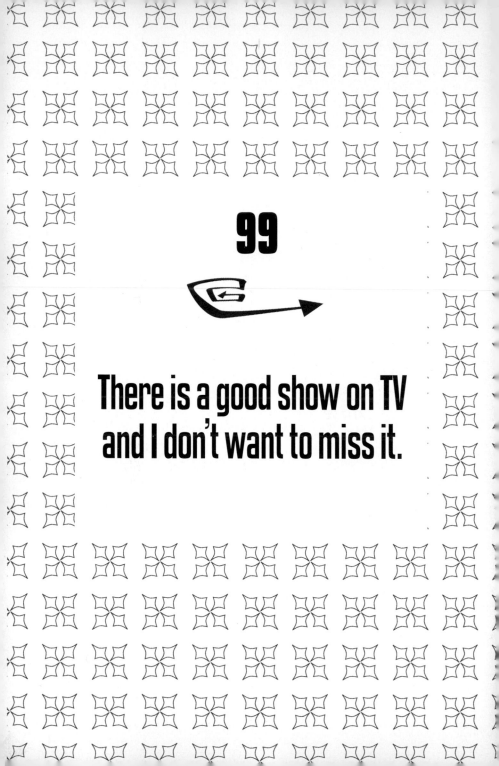

There is a good show on TV and I don't want to miss it.

Buy a stationary bike or treadmill for your home and stick it in front of your TV.

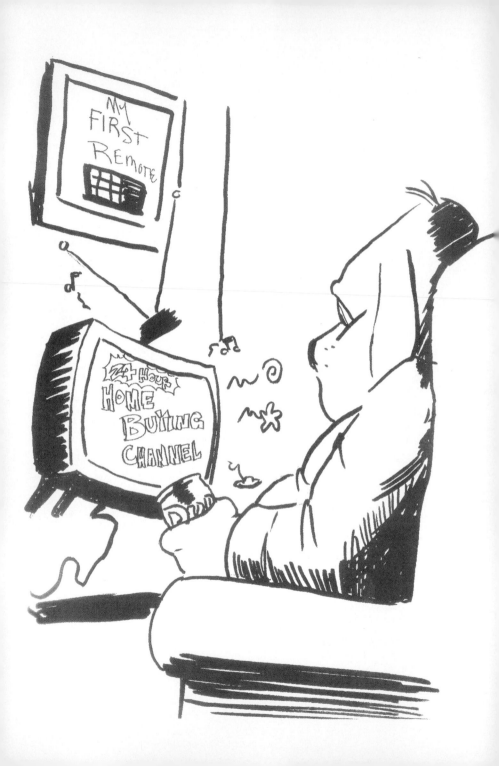

Take your TV with you. Nowadays, you can. Sony™ makes a Watchman™ portable television that can be held in your hand. You may be able to walk in only one direction, though, to get good reception (just kidding). It is difficult to see your surroundings if you are watching a TV, so walk in a quiet area where there are not too many cars or other hazards.

Exercise at a gym where there are TVs. You should have a lot of gym choices, because this is a big selling point. Some gyms allow the exercisers to have control of the channel changing, although popular programming like football and baseball games is usually shown. If you are a talk show or soap opera junkie, the majority might defeat you. Also, I have seen gym TVs where the sound is not audible unless you have a portable radio on which a particular frequency carries the sound. This is a good idea for those who do not want to have to listen to the television at all and for those who want to have control of the volume.

Buy a stationary bike or treadmill for your home and stick it in front of your TV. This way you will have total control of the programming and volume and you will not need to leave the house. You will probably find yourself exercising longer than you had planned, since you would like to finish watching a show, you might as well continue exercising. If you cannot afford a piece of equipment, walk or jog in place— just get yourself off the couch! Lastly, try muting the television during a sporting event, turning on some music, and dancing. How fun!

 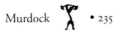

100

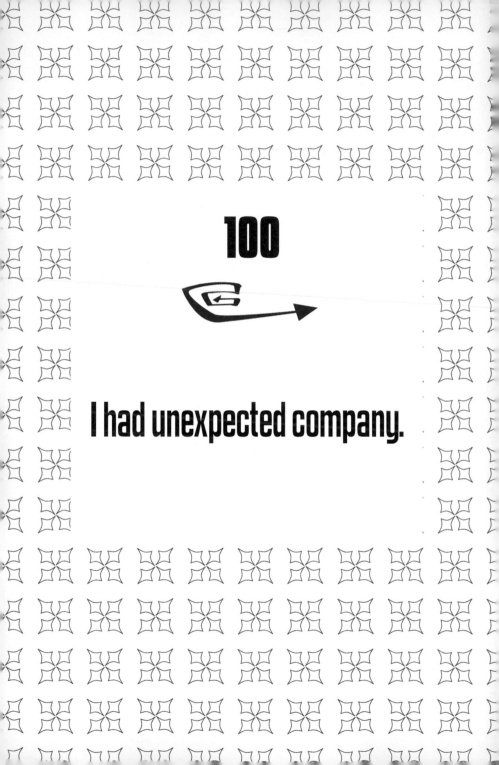

I had unexpected company.

Ya, procrastination. Or was it your Russian friend, Mr. Putitov? Was it your Ex.? Ex-cuse? Now we are getting closer to the truth.

When you have unexpected company, you have three things you can do: 1) ask them to come back after you have finished exercising, 2) ask them to join you in your workout, or 3) let them sit and talk to you while you are exercising. Did you notice that not exercising was not listed? It is not an option.

It is nice to have someone surprise you with a visit, but sometimes it is not convenient. Do not be afraid to ask friends to come back later. If they are good friends, they will not only understand, but also appreciate that you are making your health a high priority. Set a time when it would be convenient for you both to meet again.

My favorite of the three choices is to have your friend exercise with you. It is nice to have a friend be your workout partner, because you get to spend quality time together, motivate each other, and make sure that you are both maintaining compliance. Whenever one of you needs to talk, you can go for a walk instead of just sitting with the phone in your hand. You can maintain your health and friendship at the same time. Secondly, it is not uncommon to have motivation lacking at times, whether it is before or during a workout. A friend and workout partner can not only get you to the gym, but also encourage you to work hard while you are there. She can help you to exercise at your maximum potential, while still being safety conscious. It is difficult to quit an exercise program when you know that your workout partner has not. You may not want him to lose respect for you, to look better than you may, or to be more dedicated than you may. It does not matter what the reason is, just so it keeps you exercising.

You may choose to invite your company in and let them watch you exercise. If nobody minds, then everyone ends up happy. They get to visit with you and visa versa, and you get to workout. You will not be the best listener, since you will have something else taking your attention, but maybe your company will not mind.

 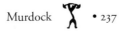

101

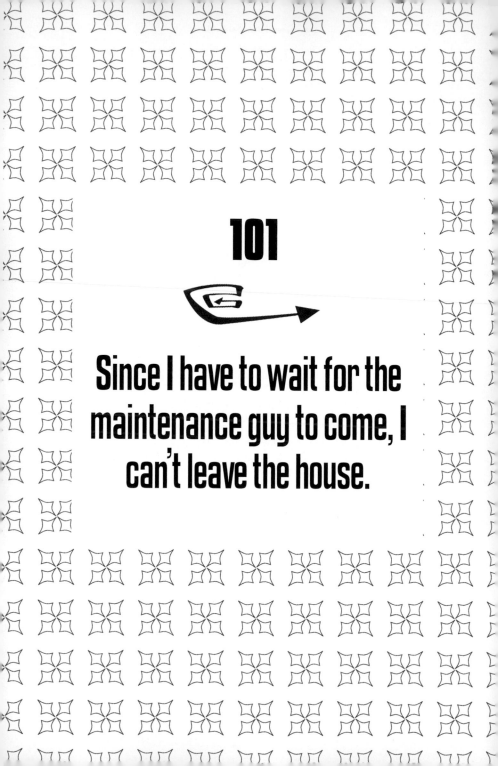

Since I have to wait for the maintenance guy to come, I can't leave the house.

You probably have a good idea of when you want to exercise, so schedule the maintenance guy to come at a different time. Make exercise a high priority instead of canceling it completely.

"When can you come fix my sink?" asks the homeowner.

"How's about Wednesday?" asks the plumber.

"Can you be a little more specific?"

"Sure. I'll be there some time between 8 a.m. and 5 p.m."

Isn't that normally the case? So, yes, I do understand that you need to stay home all day to wait for the maintenance guy, but you do not need to be sedentary all day. Take advantage of being able to get things done that will also count for exercise. Wash your car, clean the house, or do yardwork. If doing chores does not appeal to you, make up a home workout. Turn on the radio and run or walk in place or around the house or dance. Climb some stairs, jump rope or get out your kid's pogo stick (not recommended for indoor use). Using a pogo stick is a great way to burn Calories and learn balance and coordination, although it may not be for those who are concerned about falling and breaking a bone. Consult your doctor before trying a pogo stick. Lastly, remember that you do not need to be confined to your home while waiting. Walk, skate, or bike up and down your street where you can still see anyone arriving at your house.

If you are concerned about the maintenance guy calling while you are outside, change your outgoing message on your answering machine to say that you are outdoors where you cannot hear the phone. That way he will know that you are still home. You might also ask that he leave a message saying what time he expects to arrive. Then check your messages periodically.

 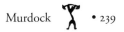

102

I'm moving and I want to wait to join a gym in my new area.

Wait, wait, wait. Why are there so many excuses that involve waiting to exercise? Why wait to feel well? In this hurry up world of ours, people have become less and less patient. To accommodate, there are expressways, supermarket express checkout stands, and express pizza delivery for example. So why wait to exercise? Let us be impatient! Let us have a workout Federal Expressed™ to us! Let us demand that Calories be burned! Do not wait. Start exercising today.

It is a good idea not to buy a membership now, if you will be moving soon. Although, some gyms offer daily, weekly, and even monthly passes. Take advantage of a short-term membership so that you know what type of gym you want to join in your new town. Will you need a gym that offers aerobics, a pool, a juice bar, or a stairclimber? The more a gym offers the more expensive it will be. Maybe you want just a basic weight room and do cardiovascular exercise outdoors. You will not know until you try.

If you already know what kind of gym you want, start exercising today and get a head start on your exercise program. Being fitter will help when it comes time to move, because your muscles will be stronger and less prone to injury. Also, some gyms require or highly recommend a fitness evaluation when you first join, so train for it. Start exercising today and attain better results on your test than you would if you had not been exercising at all. The longer you wait the harder it is to start.

 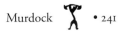

103

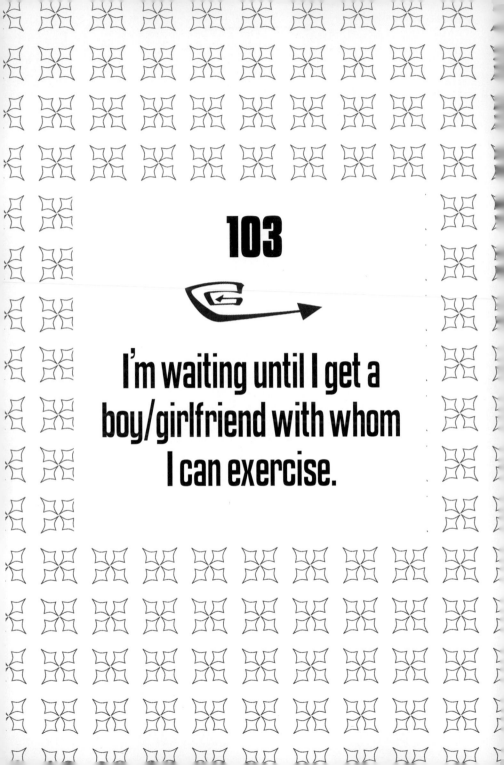

I'm waiting until I get a boy/girlfriend with whom I can exercise.

What if you never do find a mate? What if you stay single the rest of your life? Does that mean you will never exercise? Try getting a friend to be your exercise partner in the meantime.

If you are an exerciser before you meet someone, you are more marketable. People who exercise tend to look for others who do the same. Additionally, being an exerciser greatly increases the number of meeting places for "potential material":

- Take up skiing—meet someone on a ski lift.
- Take up dancing—meet someone in a class or at a nightclub.
- Take up biking—meet someone in a biking club or tour group.

Simply getting interested in sports and exercising in general should give you the motivation to sign up for a class at the local college or recreation center or to join an athletic club. In San Diego there is a club called the Athletic Singles Association. The members get together periodically and do a wide variety of exercise-related activities.

Remember one of the main reasons why people exercise in the first place: to look good! Start exercising now, while you are looking for Mr. or Miss Right, to improve your body image and to make you appear more attractive. We cannot deny that first impressions count for a lot and that clothing can cover up only so much. If you really want to find a mate, start exercising now (since you need to anyway) and you may get noticed more often.

If you start exercising now, are consistent for life, and never find a mate, at least you will have your health. That counts for a lot.

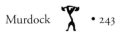

104

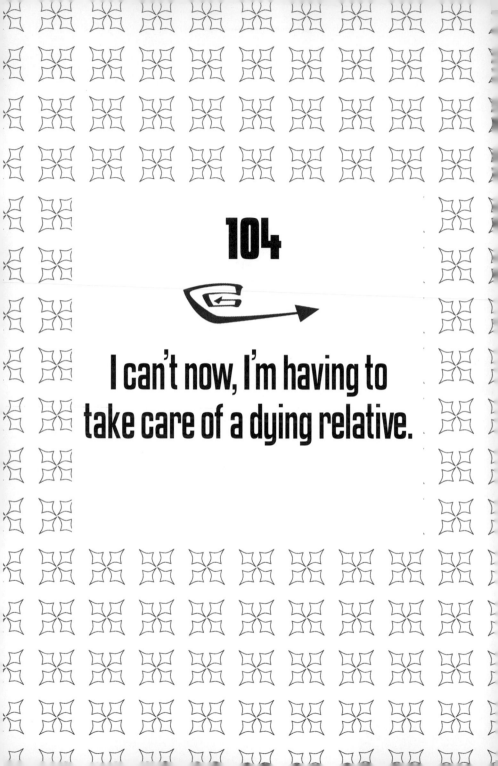

I can't now, I'm having to take care of a dying relative.

Remember to take care of your own health, too. After you relative dies, you should still have your health. Do not let it decline because you're busy being a caregiver. If you spent an hour or more exercising each day and are not doing any exercising now, you made the wrong decision. At least do the minimum of 30 minutes, five days a week. Do no completely give up exercising.

Let us review some of the benefits of excrcise and how they pertain to your caregiving.

- Stress reduction—facing the reality of death approaching soon is very stressful. Help your relative enjoy his last few days, weeks, or months, without being exposed to your anxiety. Also, you are more prone to illness if you are under stress, making you a less effective caregiver.
- Increased muscle strength—needed for helping your relative to move, pushing a wheelchair, and doing housework.
- Increased energy—gets you through the day of added responsibilities, errands, and chores. Seeing you perky may help your relative feel better. It is stressful for a patient to see the toll his disease is taking on his caregiver.
- Creativity—find ways to keep your relative busy and his mind off of his discomfort. Design games that he can play according to his potential.
- Inherited diseases—one day will you get what your relative has? Exercise can help prevent the onset of some inherited diseases like cancer.
- Sleep—do not lose sleep from worrying about your relative. Exercise can help improve sleep habits.
- Relaxation—make time not only for exercising, but also for relaxing. Exercise can help you to relax.
- Work productivity—it might be hard to concentrate on work when you are worrying about your relative. Exercise can help by improving mood state, mental awareness, and energy.

Make time for yourself. Ask for help. Have other relatives share some of the responsibilities. There are also several non-profit organizations available to help. Some provide respite, which means a person comes into the home temporarily, so that you can have a break. Hospice care is available in many areas, too, which are designed to help patients and families facing terminal illness. They provide spiritual, emotional, bereavement, physical, and social support. Some offer a nursing home or a full-time in-home nurse. Check your phone book for help in your area.

 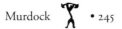

105

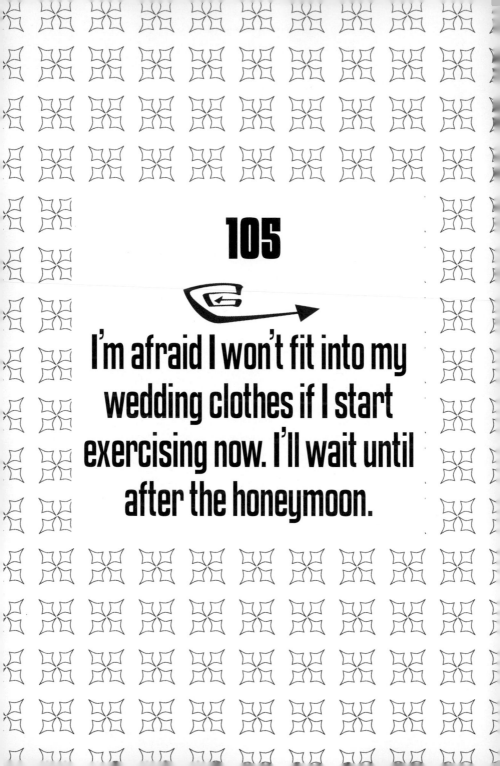

I'm afraid I won't fit into my wedding clothes if I start exercising now. I'll wait until after the honeymoon.

Start exercising now. If you are able to make that significant of a change, you can get your wedding clothes altered. If you are renting clothes, you can just get a different size. You want to look as good as possible for your wedding, anyway, right? Of course. Who wouldn't?

Not only make a commitment to each other to stay together for life, but also to exercise for life. Get your fiancée to start exercising with you today if you don't already. It will be one more thing that you will have in common and that you can do together. Really, it will be more than one thing that you can do together. There is a long list of activities that count as exercise: walking, tennis, gardening, biking, and ice skating. If your future mate does not want to start exercising and never plans to, you may have chosen the wrong person. It would be better to marry someone who wants to be healthy. What would be better: a life with someone who lives a long time without any lifestyle-related diseases or a life with someone who, from a relatively young age is dependent on your caregiving?

There is another bonus to start exercising now, besides taking care of you. You will be in better shape for your honeymoon than you would be otherwise. Having exercised for a few months, you will have a broader spectrum of things that you can do on vacation. You can go hiking, touring on bicycle, snorkeling, horseback riding, and more. If you were planning on being active anyway, you will be able to do a lot without getting tired.

106

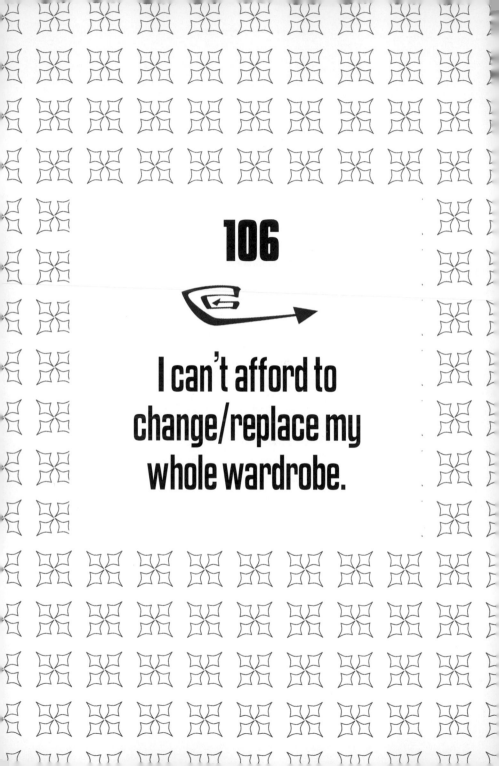

I can't afford to change/replace my whole wardrobe.

Well, I do not know what the final bill would be these days for open-heart surgery, but I bet that it is a lot more than a new wardrobe. But let's say the clothes are more expensive than the surgery. Would you rather have a healthy heart and wear clothes from Target™ or be ill and wear fancy clothes?

Why talk about open-heart surgery? As discussed earlier in the book, obesity is a risk factor for heart disease. Additionally, exercise can not only reduce body fat, but also the risk of having a heart attack. Start exercising today and lose those extra pounds. Let your body change to a healthier shape. As your clothes become looser fitting, alter them. Then, when you have reached your goal of a healthy body fat percentage (men: 10–15%, women: 15–20%), you can slowly replace your clothes with better-fitting ones. It will be nice to have new clothes, a new body, and a lower risk for cancer, heart disease, and diabetes.

For some people, having to replace a wardrobe is quite a bonus—they get to shop! Maybe, one day medical insurance companies will cover new wardrobes, knowing that the expense is less than open-heart surgery.

Even if you are not obese, exercise can change your body shape. That is OK. Keep in mind the four primary risk factors for heart disease: smoking, high blood pressure, high cholesterol, and a sedentary lifestyle. Exercising eliminates the sedentary lifestyle risk factor.

 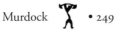

107

My spouse won't let me. He/She is afraid I'll look too good, then others will notice me more and I'll lose interest in him/her.

Maybe you should lose interest in your spouse if he is that insecure, unsupportive, and controlling. It is not right for someone to object to you exercising. I bet you can think of other cases, too, in which you were not allowed to do what you wanted. Think carefully.

Take care of yourself, by exercising, and let yourself look good. The benefits far outweigh your spouse's pessimism not to exercise. Let others notice you more often, it will make you feel great and improve your self-esteem. Self-esteem can help make you a happy person, get you the job you have always wanted, and break away from an unhealthy relationship.

If you love your spouse and you know that you two should be together, you will not lose interest in him. Try to convince him of that. He will need to accept that you are ready to take care of yourself, by exercising regularly. If it means that in addition to being healthier, more men are going to notice you, then think of it as a bonus.

Have your spouse start exercising with you. If he will not or already does by himself, maybe he should start counseling instead. He should face his personal issues that have made you neglect your health. Meanwhile, start your exercise program and take care of yourself. You will appreciate it in the future.

 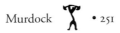

108

I have to take my pet
to the vet.

Go ahead and take your animal to the vet. While you are waiting for it to be seen, walk it in the waiting room or outside. You will get some exercise and your pet will lose some anxiety. They always seem to know when they are at the vet.

Before your pet is called into the room, ask how long the appointment will be. Then when it is your pet's turn to be seen, go for a walk outside for the duration of the appointment. Remember to tell someone at the front desk that you will be back shortly. Arrive a few minutes early, just in case the doctor is done sooner than expected. With this plan, you will not be missing your exercise for the day and you will probably be relaxed. Some pet owners have just as much anxiety as their pets do.

 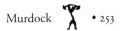

109

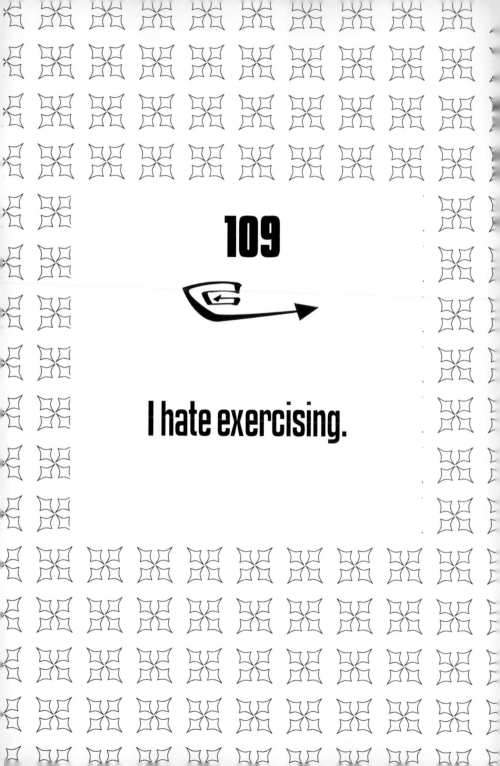

I hate exercising.

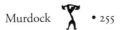

Believe me. I have heard this excuse a lot. I had a friend in college who hated exercising so much that she would not only park as close as possible to a shopping center's store, but also drive across the lot to go to another store. Needless to say, she was obese and still is. She tried to lose weight via dieting, but always gained back more weight than she had lost. Folks: DIETS DON'T WORK!

In order to fulfill your wants and needs, I bet that you do other things that you do not like doing. For instance: waiting in line at the bank so that you can have cash in your pocket or money in your account; house and clothes cleaning so that you can live hygienically; changing a child's diaper so that you are not arrested for child abuse; and waiting to be seen by a doctor so that you can have a check-up. Two things I do not like doing, but know I have to, are brushing and flossing my teeth. I do them twice and once a day, respectively, because I do not want my teeth to fall out by the time I am 45 years old. (I was born in 1968.)

Figure out what you do not like about exercising and then write it down. You will probably find that they are just additional excuses, which can be found in this book. Do you think exercise is too painful? You do not have to workout at a high intensity for it to be effective. Do you not like having sore muscles? At the onset of an exercise conditioning program, start slowly at a low intensity no matter what exercise you choose. You will reduce your chance for injury, and improve the chance of compliance. Do you not like the types of exercises you have tried in the past? Try other ones. Try as many as you can possibly imagine. Take private lessons or a class to learn a new sport or activity. It will be a great way to become healthier, improve coordination, and meet new people.

I want to know if you like being sick more than you like exercising. If you do, then do not exercise. Just let yourself go and do not take care of yourself. Go ahead and lead an unhealthy lifestyle and risk an early, and maybe even painful, death. Being healthy takes effort, so if you want it, work for it. To be well you need to exercise, eat healthy foods, avoid smoking, and drink in moderation. For men that means at most two drinks per day, and for women it's at most one per day. (1 drink = 1 oz. hard alcohol, 4 oz. wine, 12 oz. beer). You should also control stress, and keep blood pressure and cholesterol within healthy limits ($< 140/90$ mm/Hg and < 200 mg/dl, respectively). Taking care of yourself is no guarantee against illness, but it sure helps. Review the benefits of exercise listed in the beginning of the book to remember why you need to do it, even when you hate it.

110

Exercising is against my religion.

Time to change religions. Time to convert. That is like saying that your religion does not allow you to take care of yourself. Does your religion want you to die young, so that you will visit your God soon?

Religious beliefs are based on how you interpret your religion's literature. Maybe you are interpreting it incorrectly. Religion was not designed for you to follow exactly 100%. It is important for you to make some of your own decisions and decide what is best for you. That is why we all have the ability to think logically.

Now think logically about exercise. Exercise now and exercise for life.

 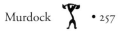

111

I got half-way to the gym, realized I left the iron on, got home, and decided not to go out again.

First, figure out a way not to let this happen again. Leave yourself a note by the front door, reminding you to turn off all appliances before leaving the house. Plan your time well so that you do not have to rush out of the house. Rushing always seems to result in something forgotten.

Secondly, as soon as you remember about the iron, see if someone else can turn it off for you. Is there a neighbor who is home and has one of your keys? Do you have a key hidden that he could use? Is there a roommate or family member who will be home, soon? You could leave him a message. Do you have a friend who could stop by your house?

Thirdly, if you must go home, do go out again. Do not punish yourself by missing your workout. By this time you will need it more than ever. You probably were stressed about the possibility of your house burning. As discussed several other times in this book, exercise can help combat stress, so let it. Go to the gym and exercise so that you do not feel guilty and stressed.

Fourth, if you are determined not to go to the gym, at least be determined to exercise. Exercise at or around your home by climbing stairs, going for a walk, bicycling, skating, dancing, or doing yardwork. You are probably already dressed for it, so go! Better yet, bring your iron with you, so that you will not have to worry about it being on.

 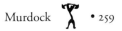

112

I'm building a house, which is taking all of my time.

Leonard Cohen in *Famous Blue Raincoat* said:

"I hear that you're building Your house deep in the desert. Are you living for nothing now? I hope you're keeping Some kind of record."

Some houses take years to build and that does not even include the planning stage or finishing touches. Does that mean you will not be exercising no matter how long it takes to build you house? You will not be exercising for a few months or years?

If you had already been exercising and then stopped, you made a big mistake. You should plan on starting from scratch once your house is finished, because you will have lost cardiovascular and muscular endurance, muscle strength, and flexibility. I am sure you remember how difficult (mentally and physically) it is to start an exercise program, so do not stop. Do not lose what you worked so hard to get.

If you had not been exercising before you started to build you house and are waiting until it is finished, you are making a big mistake. Do not put your health on hold, you might not be well when your house is finished. What good does it do to have a new house, if you cannot enjoy it? Take care of yourself now by exercising. Really enjoy your house when it is done. Remember that exercise can help you combat the stress you might be feeling now, and even prevent you from perceiving the project as being stressful.

Since your house is taking all of your time, you must not be working. Take advantage of getting to help with the house and use it as a form of exercise. Ask to do some of the physical labor like carrying wood, moving tiles, or digging dirt. After a short time of truly helping, you will realize why construction workers are in such good shape. Although, if you question why they do not all look good, your answer lies in their lunch boxes.

 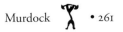

113

I hurt myself
exercising wrong.

This is why it is a good idea to use a personal fitness trainer at the start of a program. You will not only learn the best exercises for you to do, but also receive supervision to make sure that you are doing the exercises correctly. As you may realize, form is very important. Good form can help prevent injuries and lead you to your goal effectively.

I have been in many gyms where a lot of people, including body builders, are doing their exercises improperly. You cannot observe a "hard body" and think that since he looks good he must be doing the exercise properly or that you should be doing it too. Someone may look good on the outside, but what do they look like on the inside? When I see improper form, I imagine disks (between each vertebra) bulging ("slipping"), ligaments being overstretched, and muscles getting microscopic tears. I also imagine how much better they would look if they used proper form.

Some exercises are advanced, because they either take a lot of coordination and balance (which improves after a few months of exercising), or require other muscles to be strong already to stabilize non-moving joints. Don't try advanced exercises at the start of an exercise program.

Let us consider what else it takes to look as good as some of those people. Remember that diet is a factor. Body builders do not necessarily have the healthiest diets. The people that compete have diets that are extremely low in fat (yes, there is such a thing as too low) and even low in water to dehydrate themselves right before a competition. Also, anabolic steroids are used, which build muscle mass and strength when combined with exercise (35,43). They are not safe, though, with side effects including liver failure, sterility, masculinization in women, disruption of normal growth pattern, voice changes, and acne (12). Make the most of yourself without drugs. Eat a healthy diet instead.

Do not give up on exercise completely. Now that you are injured, decide how you can still exercise. This is a good time to choose a trainer. If he can safely work around your injury and motivate you not to quit, you have found a good one. Let him help you now while you are injured and later when you are healthy. It is not required that you have a trainer for life in order to be healthy, but let him put you on the right track and teach you proper form. Do not give up! You can do it! You deserve it!

 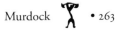

114

I just don't feel like it.

It is too bad we cannot say, "I just don't feel like getting an illness," and not contract one. We can say, "I just don't feel like exercising," and not do it, but those who say it are sure to pay for it later. How? Well, it could be in the form of a heart attack, cancer, or osteoporosis. Or, how would you like to lose your eyesight? You might if you are overweight and therefore at risk for type 2 diabetes. When glucose levels are high, damage can occur to certain body parts including the retina (the eyes' inner coat, containing nerves that connect to the optic nerve). Extensive damage to the retina will cause blindness. Thin, sedentary individuals can also develop type 2 diabetes.

Not feeling like exercising can lead you to a life of dependency. Exercising not only helps maintain your strength, but also increases it. If you do not exercise now, you eventually may depend on others to open jars, to bathe you, to get you out of a chair, and to help you walk —all tasks that you may take for granted now. Do not sit back and watch yourself lose your independence when you do not have to. It is never too late to start, so feel like it now!

The more you exercise the more you will feel like it. How exercise will make you feel and the results that you will see will keep you coming back for more. The more you exercise the more results you will obtain. It is a cyclical effect! You have nothing to lose except . . . weight.

115

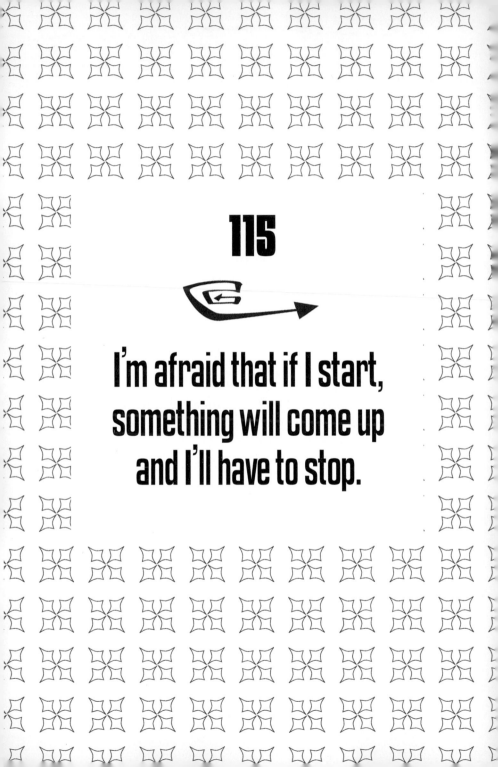

I'm afraid that if I start,
something will come up
and I'll have to stop.

Dr. Robert Schuller asked:

"What would you attempt to do if you knew you could not fail?"

Do not be afraid. We need to take chances in life or else we do not get much of what we want. If you went to college, you took a chance of either getting a degree or flunking school. You thought the benefits of having a degree were too great not to try for it. If you bought a lottery ticket, you took a chance of either winning millions of dollars or losing one dollar. You thought that the benefits of having the money were greater than losing one dollar. Start exercising and take the chance that either you will reach your goal or make an excuse to stop. Teach yourself to think that the benefits of exercising are too immensely important not to do it, because they are.

We need to make decisions or else we defeat the purpose of having choices. If we did not make decisions everyday determining what we will eat, we would starve. If we all chose not to vote on who would lead our country, we would have a dictatorship. Without further consideration, make the decision now to start exercising today. Do not fear failure. If I were afraid of failure, I would not have gone to college, started a business, or written this book.

"Courage atrophies from lack of use."
                                                    --unknown

This book was written to illustrate that you do not have to stop exercising. No matter what your excuse is, besides being sick, there is always some way you can still exercise. Even if you do get sick, you can exercise when you feel better. I am sure there will be some unexpected life event that will arise, but you will not have to stop exercising. In fact, exercise may help you get through the events. Remember that no one can make you stop. So, start now and prove it to yourself that you are in charge of your life.

 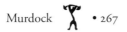

116

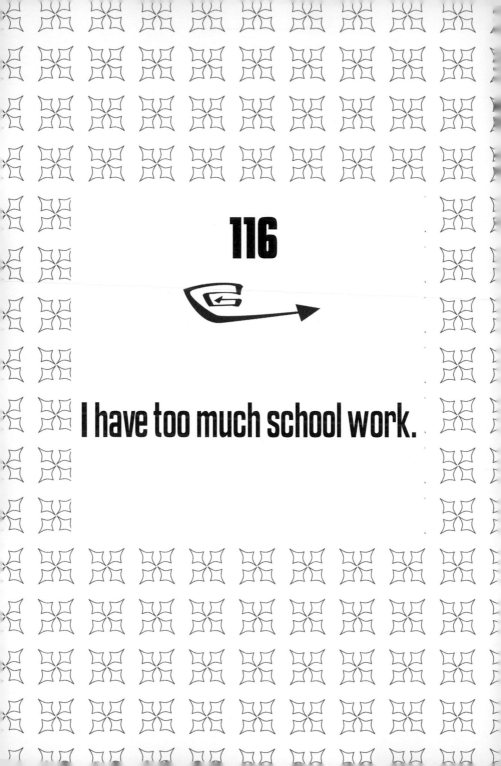

I have too much school work.

Believe me. I know what it is like to have too much schoolwork. I also know that exercise helped keep my sanity and concentration for studying. To be in control again, I exercised when I was feeling overwhelmed with homework. Also, to regain a clear, calm mind, I exercised when I started feeling spaced out.

It is a great study break, because after a few hours everything starts to look the same, and seems to be without meaning. All of the math equations, textbooks' words, and computer images start to look alike. After a few minutes of raising your heart rate, though, you can regain comprehension. Have you tried studying with your eyes at half-staff? Take a study break of exercise to wake up. Walk, bike, stairclimb, do aerobics to a video, or jog in place or around the room. It works. An exercise study break is also good for those of you who tend to overeat while studying, whether it is because you think that eating helps you learn or that eating helps ease your nerves. Whatever the reason, exercise helps to curb your appetite so that you will not be overweight by the time you have finished school.

Do not wait until you are done with school to start exercising. If you are in grade school and are waiting until you get to college, you will be in for a big surprise. You will be getting more work, not less. If you are in college and are waiting until you graduate, you are in for a shocker, too. You will not be less busy than you are now; it will just be a different kind of busy. Start exercising now, for life. Do not put it off, because it is just as important as your school work if not more so. Remember that this is your health we are discussing. What good are intelligence and an education if you do not have your health? You will not be around to use what you have learned, if you do not take care of yourself now.

 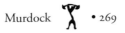

117

It's too boring.

It does not have to be. "Individuals should be encouraged to monitor the amount of enjoyment they derive from their activity, and to take responsibility for making it more enjoyable, if it is not currently meeting their needs" (5). If you have a personal fitness trainer or a gym membership, it is your responsibility to tell someone that you are bored with your program and it is her job to give you a new environment, goal, partner or group, or activity. There are too many activities and settings available these days for you to be bored. Maybe you need to have a variety of activities in each session. Maybe you like one activity, but you are bored with the environment in which it is conducted. Change it! You need to exercise for the rest of your life, so you might as well find a variety of exercises that you enjoy.

Try adding competition to relieve boredom. If you like to walk, sign up for a 5K (3.1 miles) or a 10K (6.2 miles) walk. There are many offered, usually to raise money for a non-profit organization, like the American Heart Association. You would be taking care of yourself and others by raising money. Consider fun runs, or more competitive races like half-marathons or marathons. They would not only be quite an accomplishment, but also be another reason to stick with your routine. There are also events for those of you who like to bike, skate, and swim. Join a class or a team and meet people who like to do the same activity as you. Call your local junior college, YMCA/YWCA, or recreation department for more information.

118

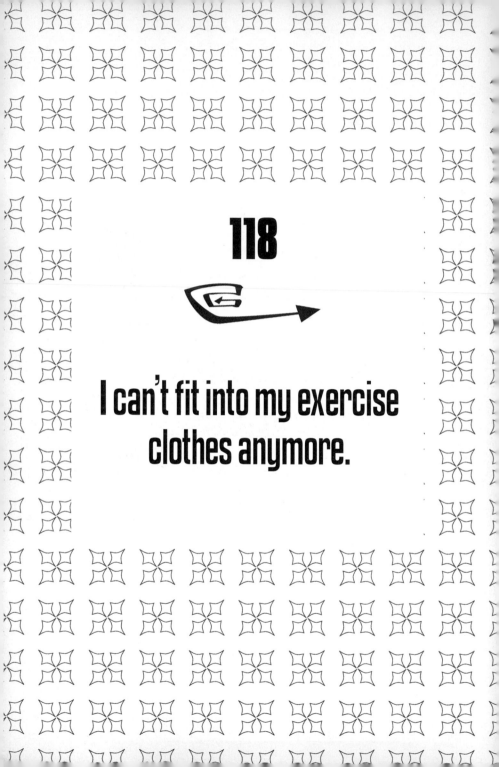

I can't fit into my exercise clothes anymore.

Go out and buy some new clothes, if you are determined to have something special in which to exercise.

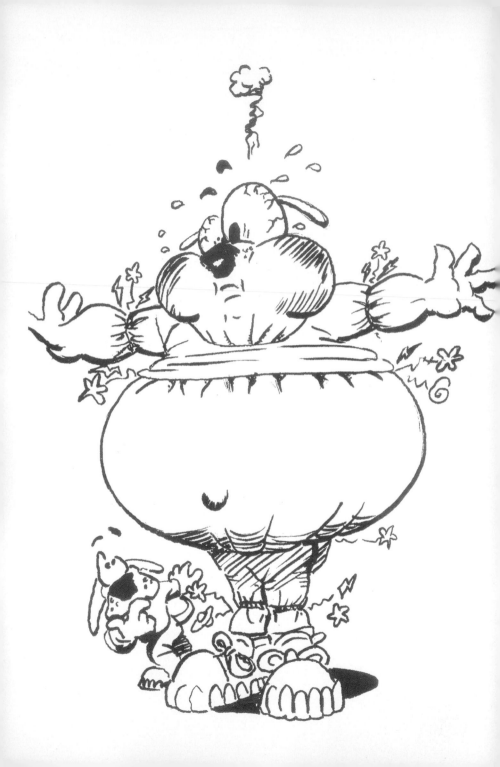

You do not have to wear special clothes to exercise. They just need to be comfortable. If you do not have any comfortable clothes, you may want to re-evaluate your wardrobe. Why wear what you do, if it does not fit right?

Go out and buy some new clothes, if you are determined to have something special in which to exercise. It does not have to be anything fancy like a leotard or running tights—just comfortable. Do not bother buying too many or ones that are too expensive, because they will not fit eventually, right? Right. Think positively! You will reach your goal and you will be able to wear your old exercise clothes, again. In fact, having your old clothes nearby may motivate you to start exercising for life.

Although for some of you, giving away your old exercise clothes after buying new ones may be the right thing to do. You may be trying to hurry to fit into them again when weight loss should be done slowly to be most effective. Being in a hurry can lead to drastic actions like dieting and overexercising. Take your time and do it right. Besides, how old are those outfits, anyway? Realistically, will you ever be that size again? Think about it. Are the clothes 5, 10, 20, 30 years old? Having a goal of wearing those clothes again may not be a healthy one. Additionally, you will just get frustrated when you try on the clothes and they still do not fit. If the clothes have not been worn in over 10 years, get rid of them. They are probably out of style anyway. Get rid of the old clothes and use new clothes as a reward to yourself each time you become a smaller size.

 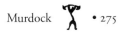

119

I have jet lag.

Jet lag has been studied, but not a lot. We know that it is more prevalent when one flies east rather than west, especially when more than two time zones are crossed.

"Jet lag occurs because the brain's biological clock, which controls the sleep/wake cycle, remains set at the time back home. Its wearisome symptoms disappear only after the clock has gradually reset itself, cued by new sunrise, sunset and living schedules" (19).

The reason why jet lag is not a valid excuse is because we can alleviate the symptoms with exercise. According to Wesley Seidel, director of the Center for Insomnia Research at Stanford University Medical School, one should walk in the morning after flying east and in the late afternoon after traveling west to reset one's clock. It is thought that the sunlight can help, too (19).

You can help avoid jet lag. If you are visiting an area for only a day or two, stay on your usual sleep/wake schedule. If you are staying for a longer time, get right into the new routine. Avoid alcohol because it dehydrates the body, hindering its ability to adjust properly.

 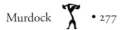

120

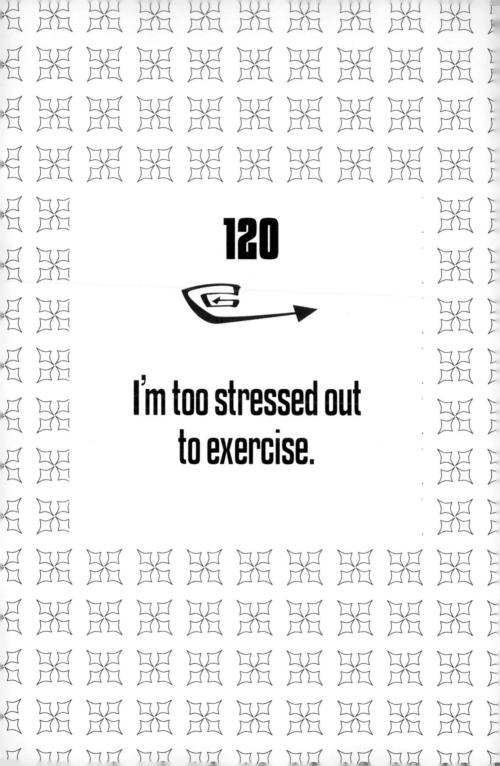

I'm too stressed out to exercise.

Dr. Albert Ellis said:

Practically all human misery and serious emotional turmoil are quite unnecessary—not to mention unethical. You, unethical? When you make yourself severely anxious or depressed, you are clearly acting against you and are being unfair and unjust to yourself.

That is even more reason to exercise. Many studies have demonstrated the effects of exercise on mental health, including stress. "'The effects are most obvious immediately after a workout and can last for several hours,' says psychologist Thomas Plante at Santa Clara (Calif.) University. Even more important, long-term exercisers seem to possess an overall sense of well-being that extends into other areas of their lives. Dr. Nieman found that after six weeks, the walkers in his study were significantly less stressed than the sedentary women" (9). It is thought that the calming effect is due to a core temperature increase that occurs during vigorous exercise. When the body gets to about 100° F (98.6° F is normal) this tranquilizing effect is produced.

Stress hormones such as cortisol and epinephrine are released during vigorous exercise to prepare the body for fight or flight. As you exercise more consistently, it is easier to handle anxiety-related events, because the body reacts less intensely to stress. It is also thought that exercise can help the body eliminate stress-related hormones to detoxify itself (1). The cause may be an increased metabolic level during exercise.

There are three other theories that give a possible explanation to exercise's effect on stress. "One states that physical training gives people a sense of mastery or control over themselves and their environment. This feeling of control becomes associated with a sense of well-being that enhances self-concept and self-efficacy, reduces anxiety and positively affects other personality variables" (29), according to Greist et al (21).

Another similar theory is that depression and anxiety can be relieved by an altered state of mind. In other words, exercise is a type of meditation (46).

Exercise seems to enable one to adapt better to the environment. When one exercises, autonomic responses (heart rate and blood pressure) are slowed thereby decreasing body tumult (agitation) (18).

 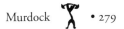

Conclusion

Besides certain illnesses, there is no valid excuse not to exercise. Reap the advantages of exercise listed in the introduction, by taking three steps: 1) understand why you formulate excuses, 2) compare them to the benefits of exercise, and 3) learn to discard the excuses. If you can take all three steps, you will be a consistent and compliant exerciser for life! Imagine experiencing all 101 benefits!

When driving the highway to wellness, steer clear of health quackery—false or misleading claims. If a product or service advertises fast or easy-to-obtain results, the fountain of youth, or a fixed-term program, it will not work. As for exercise, no effective weight loss program provides such choices. The road to wellness has no finish line; it extends until death. Pull over to heed necessary rest stops, do not exit, and be considerate to others. After all, some others contribute to laying new road. You would not want them to run out of asphalt, would you?

I would like to give you sample exercises to perform at home or in a gym that will assist you in achieving good health, but I do not know enough about you. As discussed earlier, many videotapes and books market the perfect workout. Even if the author of a videotape or book is credible, he cannot possibly give you a personalized program without knowing you! Remember that these are mass-produced items. Do you really think that there are thousands of people with the same exercise goals and the same medical history as you? These are the facts that a personal fitness trainer needs to consider.

After obtaining your physician's approval to commence an exercise program, consult a personal fitness trainer in your area. He should hold at least a Bachelor of Science degree in an exercise-related field. This route should be taken to get your personalized workout.

* * *

The clock ticks, approaching that magic hour—5:00 p.m. You are thinking, "Right after work, my exercise program commences. Goodbye, weight. Hello, waist line."

With fifteen seconds to go to freedom, the boss bellows, "By the way, there's a meeting after work today. I'll see you in 30 minutes."

"That's OK. I'll workout after the meeting."

Bingo! *That* is the attitude you should have. Now put your excuses aside and treat yourself to a healthy lifestyle. You deserve it!

 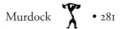

Glossary (13,15,41,45)

Activated charcoal: Medicine used in various forms of poisonings.

Anaerobic (Lactate) threshold: The point at which, during exercise, the body can not keep up with the muscles' demand for oxygen. Therefore, glucose (sugar) metabolizes without oxygen, resulting in a substrate called lactate (lactic acid).

Anemia: A blood condition, usually marked by too few red blood cells.

Asthmatics (Asthma): Narrowing of lung airways, varying over short periods of time.

Asymptomatic: Without symptoms. A symptom is subjective (immeasurable, like a headache) evidence that someone is sick.

Basal metabolic rate (BMR): The speed at which Calories are burned during sleep—the time when the least amount of energy is expended.

Blood plasma: The fluid portion of the circulating blood.

Blood pressure: The amount of force exerted against blood vessel walls during the contracting and resting phases of the heartbeat.

Calorie(s): A calorie (notice the lower case "c") is the amount of energy it takes to raise 1 milliliter of water at 15° Celsius by 1° Celsius. A Calorie or kilocalorie (kcal) is 1000 calories. Nutritional literature and food labels refer to Calorie. For example, a medium apple contains 80 Calories (kcals).

Cancer: A group of diseases characterized by abnormal, uncontrolled growth of body cells.

Cardiac reserve: The mechanisms available to the heart in its adjustment to supply the oxygen needs of exercised muscle tissue.

Cardiovascular exercise: Continuous, rhythmic movement of large muscle groups (e.g., legs and/or arms) at an intensity of 60%-90% of maximum heart rate for at least five minutes.

Carpal tunnel syndrome: Pain, tingling, burning, and numbness in the hand caused by compression of a nerve in the wrist.

Cartilage: Connective tissue, usually found in joints.

Cervix: The lower part of the uterus that extends into the vagina.

Chemotherapy: Mostly used in cancer patients. The treatment is by means of chemical substances or drugs.

Circadian rhythm: The biologic variations with a cycle of about 24 hours.

Colon: The large intestines.

Dehydration: Not having enough water.

Diabetes: Type 2 (non-insulin dependent): Usually starts in adulthood, due to heredity and/or obesity. Since obesity in children is on the rise, type 2 diabetes is being diagnosed at younger and younger ages. When diabetes strikes, the body's cells become insensitive to insulin. Type 1 (insulin-dependent): Usually starts by the age of 20, marked by the inability to produce insulin.

Diet(s): A particular way of eating. This term usually denotes a reduction in Calories to lose weight.

Dumbbells: Hand-held weights, used for strength training exercises.

Endometriosis: The formation of cysts, usually, of the uteral (uterus) lining.

Endorphins: The body's natural painkiller.

Excuse(s): To release from an obligation or duty.

Exercise: Bodily exertion for the sake of restoring the organs and functions to a healthy state or keeping them healthy.

Fetal (fetus): Represents the product of conception from the end of the eighth week of pregnancy

 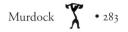

to the moment of birth.

Glucose tolerance: The ability to use blood sugar.

HDL (high-density lipoprotein) cholesterol: HDL is known as the "good" cholesterol. It carries fat away from the arteries to the liver where it can be excreted via bile (aids in digestion).

Heart disease: The inability of the heart and/or blood vessels to maintain proper blood flow, and to deliver oxygen to the body's tissues.

Heat exhaustion: A milder form of heatstroke, marked by cool, clammy skin. The condition should still be taken seriously, though, and the patient should be treated with a cool bath or ice packs.

Heatstroke: A severe illness produced by exposure to excessively high temperatures and characterized by headache, dizziness, confusion, and a slight rise in body temperature. In severe cases, collapse and coma occur, preceding hot dry skin.

Heimlich Maneuver: Used to clear an obstructed airway of a choking victim. Call the American Red Cross or the American Heart Association to learn how to perform it.

Hypertension: High blood pressure. A value > 145/95 mm/Hg.

Immune system: Tries to keep us free from invading organisms such as bacteria and viruses that may cause diseases.

Insulin: A hormone produced by the pancreas to promote glucose utilization, protein synthesis, and the formation and storage of fat.

Intrauterine: Within the uterus (where a baby develops).

Ipecac Syrup: Used to induce vomiting, after poisoning.

Lactic acid: A substrate when glucose is metabolized without oxygen.

LDL (low-density lipoprotein) cholesterol: LDL is known as the "bad" cholesterol. It delivers cholesterol to the arteries, where it is then deposited in the walls.

Ligaments: Connect bone to bone.

Maximum oxygen uptake ($\dot{V}O_2$ max): The most amount of oxygen that the cells can use. It is measured in milliliters of oxygen per minute per kilogram of body weight (ml/min/kg).

Menstrual (Menstruation): The shedding of the uteral (uterus) lining at the beginning of a woman's cycle. Cycles are typically 28 days long.

Myocardial infarction: Heart attack. Death of heart tissue, from lack of oxygen to it.

Obese: Having too much body fat. In men: more than 25% body fat. In women: more than 30% body fat.

Osteoarthritis: Degenerative joint disease. Very common in older persons, especially affecting weight-bearing joints. Articular (joint) cartilage becomes soft, frayed, and thinned.

Osteoporosis: Reduction in the quantity of bone, resulting in porous, brittle bones.

Palpitations: Forcible pulsations of the heart.

Personal fitness trainer: One who administers fitness evaluations and prescribes exercise programs. Some consult nutritionally, too.

Polio: Poliomyelitis. Inflammation of the gray matter of the spinal cord, caused by an acute, infectious disease. Can cause paralysis (loss of muscle function) and even death. Thanks to Dr. Salk, a vaccine exists.

Polypropylene: A synthetic material in clothing, effective in keeping moisture away from the skin.

Postpartum: After childbirth.

Prenatal: Preceding childbirth.

 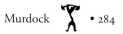

Prostate: A gland found only in men, located just below the bladder. It secretes an alkaline fluid, discharged with semen.

Pulmonary: Relating to the lungs.

Reflux: Indigestion. Heartburn. A backward flow of stomach acid.

Respiratory tract: The path leading from the nose into the lungs.

Resting metabolic rate (RMR): The speed at which Calories are burned when one is at rest.

Rosacea: Adult acne.

Shin splints: An idiopathic (of unknown origin) pain between the knee and the ankle. They can be found in one who either misuses (weekend warrior) or overuses (a high-mileage runner) exercise. It is thought that the pain derives from swelling of tibial (shin) muscles.

Shunted: Bypassed or diverted.

Side stitch: A sharp pain in the side during exercise. Still not a well-understood phenomenon, but is thought to be the result of abdominal ligaments being jarred.

Strength training: The type of exercise used to increase muscle mass, endurance, and strength.

Stressed (Stress): The reactions to forces of various abnormal states that tend to disturb the physiologic equilibrium (balance).

Stretching: Movements used to increase flexibility, range of motion, and agility.

Stroke: Lack of oxygen to one section of the brain, resulting in tissue death.

Tendons: Connect muscle to bone.

Tonicity: Usually relating to muscles. The state of continuous activity or tension beyond that related to the physical properties.

Triglycerides: A type of fat made up of one glycerol molecule and three fatty acids.

Trimester: The first, second, or third three months of pregnancy.

Type 1 & 2 diabetes: see Diabetes

Vagina: The genital canal in the female, extending from the uterus to the outside.

Viscosity: Thickness. The resistance of a fluid to flow, due to a shearing force.

Yo-yo dieting: Going on and off low-Calorie eating programs, which cause weight fluctuations.

References

1. Allen RJ. *Human Stress: Its Nature and Control.* New York: Macmillan Publishing Company, 1983.

2. American College of Obstetricians and Gynecologists. *Exercise During Pregnancy and the Postpartum Period.* Technical Bulletin #189. Washington, DC, 1994.

3. American College of Sports Medicine. *Guidelines for Exercise Testing and Prescription.* Philadelphia: Lea & Febiger, 1991.

4. American College of Sports Medicine. *Guidelines for Exercise Testing and Prescription.* Philadelphia: Lea & Febiger, 1995.

5. American College of Sports Medicine. *Resource Manual for Guidelines for Exercise Testing and Prescription.* Philadelphia: Lea & Febiger, 1988.

6. Ammons RB. Le Mouvement. In G. H. Steward and J. P. Steward (Eds.), *Current Psychological Issues.* New York: Holt, Rinehart & Winston, 1958.

7. Appenzeller O. *Sports Medicine.* Baltimore Munich: Urban & Schwarzenberg, 1988.

8. Astrand P-O, Kaare R. *Textbook of Work Physiology.* New York: McGraw Hill Book Company, 1970.

9. Chollar S. The Psychological Benefits of Exercise. *Am Health.* 1995;June:73-75.

10. Couzens GS. Toxic Workouts. *Am Health.* 1994;July/August:95-96.

11. DeBusk RF, et al. Training Effects of Long Versus Short Bouts of Exercise. *Am J Cardio.* 1990;65:1010-1013.

12. deVries HA. *Physiology of Exercise.* Dubuque: Brown and Benchmark, 1986.

13. deVries HA. *Physiology of Exercise.* Dubuque: Brown and Benchmark, 1994.

14. Dunham P. Effect of Practice Order on the Efficiency of Bilateral Skill Acquisition. *Res Quar.* 1977;48:254-287.

15. Ehrlich E, Flexner SB, Carruth G, Hawkins JM. *Oxford American Dictionary.* New York: Oxford University Press, 1980.

16. Elliott D. Manual Asymmetrics in the Performance of Sequential Movements by Adolescents and Adults with Down's Syndrome. *Am J Mental Def.* 1985;90:90-97.

17. Flippin R. Winterize Your Exercise. *Am Health.* 1994;December:80.

18. Folkins CH, Sine WE. Physical Fitness Training and Mental Health. *Am Psych.* 1981;36:373-389.

19. Gilman L. Shedding Light on Jet Lag. *Am Health.* 1989;June:46.

20. Griest JH. Exercise Intervention with Depressed Outpatients. *Exercise and Mental Health.* New York: Hemisphere, 1987.

21. Greist JH, et al. Running Through Your Mind. *J Psychosomatic Res.* 1978;22:259-294.

22. Hedley AA, Ogden CL, Johnson CL, Carroll MD, Curtin LR, Flegal KM. Prevalence of Overweight and Obesity among U. S. Children, Adolescents, and Adults. *J Am Med Assoc.* 2004;291:2847-2850.

23. Hicks RE, Gualtieri CT, Schroeder SR. Cognitive and Motor Components of Bilateral Transfer. *Am J Psych.* 1983;96:223-228.

24. Huey L, Forster R. *The Complete Waterpower Workout Book.* New York: Random House, 1993.

25. Iknoian T. What Ails Women Athletes. *Am Health.* 1993;October:55.

26. Kase LM. Understand Your Body Clock. *Am Health.* 1995;July/August:54-59.

 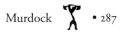

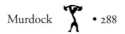

27. Kavanagh T, Shephard RJ. The Effects of Continued Training on the Aging Process. *Annals NY Acad Sci.* 1977;301:656-670.

28. Kohl RM, Roenker DL. Bilateral Transfer as a Function of Mental Imagery. *J Motor Behavior.* 1980;12:197-206.

29. Kravitz L. Exploring the Mysteries of Exercise. *IDEA Today.* 1995;January:48-55.

30. Kuczmarski RJ, et al. Increasing Prevalence of Overweight Among U. S. Adults. *J Am Med Assoc.* 1994;272:205-211.

31. Laszlo JI, Baguley RA. Motor Memory and Bilateral Transfer. *J Motor Behavior.* 1971;3:235-240.

32. Los Angeles Times. April 19, 1991.

33. Martinsen EW. Physical Exercise and Depression: Clinical Experience. *Acta Psychiatrica Scandinavia.* 1994;377:23-27.

34. Noble BJ, Borg GAV, Jacobs I, Ceci R, Kaiser P. A Category-ratio Perceived Exertion Scale: Relationship to Blood and Muscle Lactates and Heart Rate. *Med Sci Sports Ex.* 1983;15:523-528.

35. Papanicolaou GN, Falk EA. General Muscular Hypertrophy Induced by Androgenic Hormone. *Science.* 1938;83:238-239.

36. Pearl B. *Getting in Shape.* Shelter Publications, 1994.

37. Petruzzello SJ, Landers DM. State Anxiety Reduction and Exercise: Does Hemispheric Activation Reflect Such Changes? *Med Sci Sports Ex.* 1994;26:1028-1035.

38. Raglin JS. Anxiolytic Effects of Exercise. *Physical Activity and Mental Health.* Washington, DC: Francis Publishers (in press).

39. Raglin J. Exercise and Mental Health. *IDEA Today.* 1995;July/August:60-70.

40. Sarnoff PM. *The Ultimate Spa Book.* New York: Warner Books, Inc., 1989.

41. Schifferes JJ. *The Family Medical Encyclopedia.* New York: Pocket Books, 1977.

42. Sears C. No Sweat. *Am Health.* 1993;June:88.

43. Simonson E, Kearns WM, Enzer N. Effect of Methyl Testosterone Treatment on Muscular Performance and Central Nervous System of Older Men. *J Clin Endocrin Met.* 1944;10:528-534.

44. Sonstroem RJ, Morgan WP. Exercise and Self Esteem: Rationale and Model. *Med Sci Sports Ex.* 1989;21:329-337.

45. Stedman TL. *Illustrated Stedman's Medical Dictionary.* Baltimore: Williams & Wilkins, 1982.

46. Van Andel GE. Mood, Health Locus of Control and Physical Activity. Dissertation, Indiana University, 1986.

47. Wartik N. The Truth About PMS. *Am Health.* 1995;April:64.

48. Wolfe LA, et al. Prescription of Aerobic Exercise During Pregnancy. *Sports Med.* 1989;8:273-301.

About the Author

Originally from Cupertino, CA, Jeanne studied physical education at California Polytechnic State University in San Luis Obispo. She graduated in June 1991, and then moved to Honolulu, HI, where she lived for 14 months. There, BeanFit was born February 7, 1992. Initially, the services provided included personal fitness training, nutrition counseling, health education for children, and swimming and rollerskating lessons.

Since then, BeanFit has evolved.

December 1992, Jeanne moved to San Diego, CA, where she re-started her business and lived for 11 years. February 2004, Jeanne relocated to Paso Robles, CA, where she still resides.

Jeanne has always maintained a home office, while conducting phone consultations or traveling to others' homes and businesses to provide the services.

Watching people's lives improve is obvious motivation for Murdock to continue her work, but how did the passion arise? "When I was in Brownies, I was taught to help others, like seniors crossing a street. As soon as I heard that, I was hooked. Even at the young age of five, I enjoyed seniors, so I started looking for ones that I could help across the street. I still look for them, actually," she giggles.

As for the interest in health, Murdock's influence arose from a lesson called Berkeley Health that she was taught in third grade. It included nutrition education and anatomy and taught her to value wellness. Once again, she was hooked. Immediately, she practiced what she learned, including eliminating hot dogs, bacon, and caffeinated beverages from her diet. The first time she refused to eat a hot dog at home, she told her parents that it was unhealthy. Her father responded, "Your mother wouldn't cook you anything that wasn't healthy." She thought, "Oh, if you only knew." Remember that Murdock was only eight years old at the time.

Since then, Murdock has lived a very healthy lifestyle, not to live as long as possible, but to live as well as possible. She explains that life is so exciting with so many things to do and places to see, that she wants to have the energy to do it all. "All" includes motivating others to achieve their peak wellness and to live *their* lives to the fullest.

The current services offered include nutrition counseling, professional organizing, and corporate consulting: fitness centers/trainers, food manufacturers, and tailored health education lectures.

 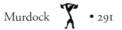

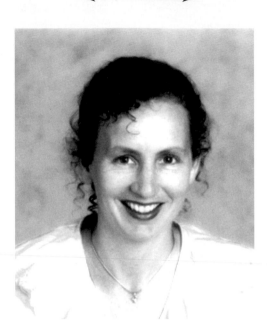

Qualifications:
- Bachelor of Science in Physical Education, concentration in Commercial / Corporate Fitness, Cal Poly State University, San Luis Obispo.
- Undergraduate Nutrition Coursework Completed, San Diego State University.
- Resource Unit, Celiac Sprue Association, San Luis Obispo County.

Memberships:
- Celiac Sprue Association
- National Association of Professional Organizers
- American Dietetic Association
- Food Allergy and Anaphylaxis Network

 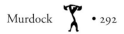

"Treat Yourself to a Healthy Lifestyle"

BEANFIT®

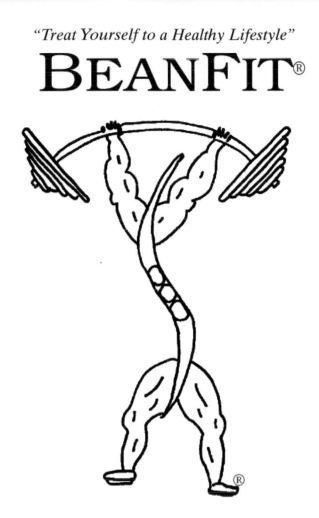

HEALTH AND FITNESS SERVICES
established 1992

Jeanne "Bean" Murdock
P.O. Box 1083
Paso Robles, CA 93447
phone/fax: 805-226-9893
www.beanfit.com
info@beanfit.com

Questions? Comments?
Please feel free to write or call Jeanne "Bean" Murdock anytime at:
BeanFit
P. O. Box 1083
Paso Robles, CA 93447
Phone/Fax: 805-226-9893
Website: www.beanfit.com
E-mail: info@beanfit.com

Visit
www.beanfit.com
for updates on new products,
including
*The Every Excuse in the Book
Calendar*

Visit
www.beanfit.com
for updates on new products,
including
The Every Excuse in the Book Calendar